OMAD DIET COOKBOOK

Copyright © 2021 by Danielle De Mayo All rights reserved. No part of this book may be reproduced in any form, either written, electronic, recording, or photocopying, without the express permission of the publisher or author. The exception would be in the case of brief quotations embodied in the critical articles or reviews and pages where the publisher or author expressly grants permission.

The quantity mentioned in recipes

1 cup =240g 0r 240ml 0r 8 ounces
1 tbsp= 15g 0r 1/2 ounce
1 tsp= 7.5g 0r 1/6 ounce

The pictures in the book do not represent precisely the recipe meal.

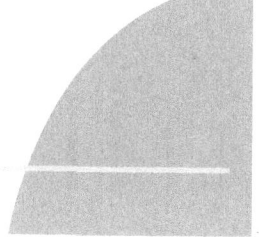

INTRODUCTION

The OMAD diet is one of the fasting diets and stands for 'One Meal A Day'. It is intermittent fasting in which you fast for 23 hours and eat for 1 hour a day. You should drink water, coffee, tea, kombucha, and other unsweet drinks during fasting hours but do not add milk or cream in coffee or tea, and do not add sugar in any other drink.

If you are eating only once a day, it is essential to eat enough different food for your proteins, fibers, vitamins, and minerals intake. In this book, you will find a 14-day meal plan to quickly start and learn how to combine different recipes in your meal.

HOW TO START

First, take one hour of your day to eat your meal in peace without stress, phone, television, etc. Eat slowly and chew and enjoy your meal.

Start your meal with low calorie fruit or vegetable salad. Remember your stomach is fasting, and eating a fatty cheeseburger as the first thing will be too heavy to digest. Listen to your body.

Always have some carrots in your fridge, so when it is time to eat and you're starving while preparing your meal, you can have a bite out of it. It is hard, and you will need to chew for a while, but it will prevent you from making yourself a fatty sandwich while you're cooking.

If you eat a big plate of pasta and hamburger in just one meal with lots of sauces and chips and no fruit and vegetables, it will not boost your energy and will be a reason why you gain weight during fasting.

When you finish your daily meal, it will be helpful to start prepping your meal for the next day, so when you are starving later, you won't need to cook and can eat right away.

RECOMMENDED FOOD

- Protein rich food like:
Meat (chicken, pork, beef), Eggs, Seafood (Fish, shells), Cheese, Tofu, Legumes

- Fat: recommanded 100 - 180 gr per day like:
Avocados, olives, olive oil, coconut oil, nuts, and any kind of seeds to be added to the meal

- Vegetables:

Carrot, broccoli, cabbage, cauliflower, beetroot, turnip, scallions, lettuce, bell peppers, sweet potato, spinach and kale spinach, Sweet potatoes, white potatoes, rice, quinoa, carrots, beetroot, turnips, mushrooms

- Fruits: Grapes, watermelon, mango, pineapple, banana etc.

- Nutrient-rich herbs and spices like dill, fennel seeds, coriander, and parsley

- You can also add fermented foods like sauerkraut and kombucha

- Any kind of bread or pasta needs to be made from whole flour, brown rice.

- Deserts made with fruit and whole flour (not refined flour), seeds, yogurt, smoothie, etc....

FOOD TO AVOID

Avoid the following food as much as you can as it will help you lose weight during your OMAD diet:
- All processed meat like sausages, hot dogs, salami, Ham, cured bacon, Salted, smoked and cured meat, fatty corned beef, dried meat, beef jerky, canned meat etc.
- Microwave popcorn
- Frozen pizza
- Fried foods like French fries, doughnuts, and fried chicken
- Non-dairy coffee creamer
- Stick margarine, shortening
- Cakes, cookies, and pies, refrigerated dough, such as biscuits and rolls, ice cream, candy, sweet beverage
- Refined carbohydrate like white bread, pizza dough, white pasta, pastries, white flour, white rice, sweet desserts, and many kinds of breakfast cereal.

BEVERAGE

Drinking a lot of fluid during your 23 hours of fasting will flush away toxins from your body and make you feel less hungry. Drinking hot beverages, like hot tea or hot coffee, will help you even more, to not feel hungry. Put a spoon or two per day of cider vinegar in your water. Or squeeze a lemon or lime in the water.

Whenever you would like to eat, drink a glass of water. You need to drink at least 2 liters of fluid a day. Do not forget to drink !! Keep the bottle with you all the time. Drinking is essential.

If you have a headache, that is probably because your body is dehydrated. Take salt and potassium supplements and plenty of fluid.

FOOD RICH IN POTASSIUM

These are some fruit and vegetables with high potassium: bananas, oranges, cantaloupe, honeydew, apricots, grapefruit, dried prunes, dried raisins, dates, cooked spinach, broccoli, potatoes, mushrooms, cucumbers, peas, zucchini, some fish like tuna, halibut, cod, and meat and poultry, nuts, brown and wild rice. These will help a lot, so include them in your meal if you have a headache.

THE POWER OF MINDSET

The second most important thing in the diet is the will. First, ask yourself why you want to start the OMAD diet. Do you want to lose weight? Why do you want to lose weight? Maybe because of health issues or you think you are not attractive? Did you recently gain some weight?

Please write down your answer and stick it on the fridge, on the kitchen door and in your room. Keep that goal in your mind all the time. Visualize yourself slimmer, healthier (if you have those problems, etc.) Keep in mind that visualization all the time.

Subscribe to a Facebook or Twitter page; those groups can inspire you. There is an excellent community outside, and you will be more than welcome.

EXERCISES

It is also essential to include some exercises in your daily routine. You can do that perhaps before your meal when your hunger starts to become more significant. At that time, you can be out on an aerobic or fitness class and forget about your hunger. You can also find plenty of exercises on the web to follow and learn.

14 - DAY MEAL PLAN

Following is the 14-day meal plan. Daily calorie intake depends on your age, height, weight, and daily activity.
You can add a few spoons of seeds or nuts to your everyday meal as they contain excellent fats. But be aware that seeds and nuts are high in calories. Per 28 gram of:

- Per 28 gram of :
- Walnuts: 183 calories
- Brazil nuts: 184 calories
- Almonds: 161 calories
- Pistachios: 156 calories
- Cashews: 155 calories
- Sunflower seeds: 164 calories
- Pumpkin seeds: 151calories
- Sesame seeds: 160calories
- Hemp seeds: 155calories
- Chia seeds: 137calories
- Flaxseeds: 152calories

14 DAYS MEAL PLAN

1ST week
Monday:
MIMOSA FRUIT SALAD	191
FALAFEL	123
GROUND BEEF AND BROCCOLI	37
ACQUACOTTA	145
COLD KIWI CREAM DESSERT	183

Tuesday:
COUSCOUS AND CHICKPEA SALAD	152
BLACK BENA MUSHROOM CHILI	115
BAKED TOFU	103
STRAWERRY MOUSSE	185

Wednesday:
HEALTY FRUIT SALAD WITH MINT CITRUS DRESSING	195
CABBAGE SOUP WITH BEEF	45
TOFU STIR FRY	101
ROASTED BEEF TANDELOIN	49
COLD KIWI CREAM DESSERT	183

Thursday:
TOMATO CUCUMBER WHITE BEAN SALAD	151
EGGLPLANT LASAGNA	131
GRILLED PORT TENDERLOIN	55
ICE CREAM SANDWICH DESSER	181

Friday:
LOW FAT FRUIT SALAD	193
PEA SPINACH CARBONARA	143
CHEESE AND BACON STUFFED MEAT PIES	93
WALNUT ROSEMARY CRUSTED SALAD	71

Saturday:
FRESH KALE SALAD WITH TAHINI DRESSING	159
VEGAN LENTIL SOUP	119
LOW CARB CHILI CHEESE FRIES	91
OVEN FRIED PORK CHOPS	59

Sunday:
GRILLED FRUIT SALAD WITH COCONUT CREAM	199
DIET PASTA	207
QUINOA STUFFED EGGPLANT WITH TAHITI SAUCE	133
PORK STIR FRY	57
SPACIED CARROT AND LENTIL SOUP	111
COLD KIWI CREAM DESSERT	183

2nd week
Monday:

TABBOULEH SALAD	157
MEDITERRANEAN LETTUCE CHICKPEA WRAPS	129
BEEF BOURGUIGNON	47
MINI FRITATAS	89

Tuesday:

MEDITERANEAN TUNNA SPINACH SALAD	155
SEED CRACKERS	121
ANUT BUTTER NOODLES WITH CRISPYPORT BELLY	53
GLUTEN FREE PASTA STYLE SALAD	165
BLUBERRY MUFFINS	171

Wednesday:

PALEO FRUIT SALAD	197
LIGHT BREAD	203
BROCCOLI AND KALE GREEN SOAP	141
GARLIC DEVIL EGGS	85
SALMON SANDWICH	65

Thursday:

BURRITOS	201
EASY BROWN RICE	209
FLAT BELLY SOUP	135
GREEN EGGS WITH SMOKED SALMON	61
LENTIL SALAD	161

Friday:

MIMOSA FRUIT SALAD	191
CHEESE AND BACON STUFFED MEAT PIES	93
MAPO TOFU	105
CHICKEN AND SPINACH SOUP	15
BULGUR SALAD WITH MARINATED FETA	163

Saturday:

TABBOULEH SALAD	157
PEA SPINACH CARBONARA	143
SWEET POTATO TOAST	147
SLOW COOKED MEDITERANEAN STEW	149
ALMOND DESSERT	179

Sunday:

MINT BASIL GRIDDLED PEACH SALAD	169
HEALTY HUMMUS	127
LIGHT BREAD	203
STEAK DINNER FOR TWO	31
CAROT PUDING	175

CONTENT

MEAT
CHICKEN
1.	Chimichurri Chicken Tray Bake	11
2.	Caprese Chicken Bowl	13
3.	Chicken and Spinach Soup	15
4.	Bacon-Wrapped Chicken Parcels	17
5.	Chipotle Chicken	19
6.	Coconut Chicken Curry	21
7.	Paillard of Chicken with Lemon and Herbs	23
8.	Lemon Parmesan Chicken with Zucchini Noodles	25
9.	Creamy Pesto Chicken Salad with Greens	27
10.	Chicken and Apple Kale Wraps	29

BEEF
1.	Steak Dinner for Two	31
2.	Steak Taco Bowl	33
3.	Corned Beef and Cabbage	35
4.	Ground Beef and Broccoli	37
5.	Mediterranean Beef and Rice	39
6.	Roasted Beef Dinner	41
7.	Hoisin Beef Noodle	43
8.	Cabbage Soup with Beef	45
9.	Beef Bourguignon	47
10.	Roasted Beef Tenderloin	49

PORK
1.	Butter Braised Cabbage with Crispy Ham	51
2.	Peanut Butter Noodles with Crispy Pork Belly	53
3.	Grilled Pork Tenderloin	55
4.	Pork Stir Fry	57
5.	Oven-Fried Pork Chops	59

FISH
1.	Green Eggs with Smoked Salmon	61
2.	Salmon Power Bowl	63
3.	Salmon Sandwich	65
4.	Creamy Pesto Tuna Salad	67
5.	Salmon and tabbouleh low carb bowl	69
6.	Walnut Rosemary Crusted Salmon	71
7.	Prawns with Pineapple and Green Beans	73
8.	Teriyaki Salmon Parcels	75
9.	Greek Shrimp Souvlaki and Farro Bowl	77
10.	Charred Shrimp Pesto Bowls	79

EGG
1. California Omelet — 81
2. Italian Egg Drop Soup — 83
3. Garlic Devil Eggs — 85
4. Spinach and Egg Scramble with Raspberries — 87
5. Mini Frittatas — 89

CHEESE
1. Low Carb Chili Cheese Fries — 91
2. Cheese and Bacon Stuffed Meat Pies — 93
3. Chaffle Sandwich — 95
4. Head Tricolore Pizza — 97
5. Mediterranean Macaroni and Cheese — 99

TOFU
1. Tofu Stir Fry — 101
2. Baked Tofu — 103
3. Mapo Tofu — 105
4. Crispy Marinated Tofu — 107
5. Crispy Baked Tofu with Bok Choy — 109

LEGUMES
1. Spiced Carrot and Lentil Soup — 111
2. Mediterranean Lentil Soup — 113
3. Black Bean Mushroom Chili — 115
4. Black Bean Tacos — 117
5. Vegan Lentil Soup — 119
6. Seed Crackers — 121
7. Falafel — 123
8. Vegan Chickpea Bowl — 125
9. Healthy Hummus — 127
10. Mediterranean Lettuce Chickpea Wraps — 129

VEGGIES
1. Eggplant Lasagna — 131
2. Quinoa Stuffed Eggplant with Tahini sauce — 133
3. Flat Belly Soup — 135
4. Cabbage Soup — 137
5. Chickpea Tomato and Spinach Curry — 139
6. Broccoli and Kale Green Soup — 141
7. Pea Spinach Carbonara — 143
8. Acquacotta — 145
9. Sweet Potato Toast — 147
10. Slow Cooker Mediterranean Stew — 149

SALADS

1.	Tomato Cucumber White Bean Salad	151
2.	Couscous and Chickpea Salad	153
3.	Mediterranean Tuna Spinach Salad	155
4.	Tabbouleh Salad	157
5.	Fresh Kale Salad with Tahini dressing	159
6.	Lentil Salad	161
7.	Bulgur Salad with Marinated Feta	163
8.	Gluten-free Pasta Style Salad	165
9.	Lemony Orzo Salad	167
10.	Mint Basil Griddled Peach Salad	169

DESSERTS

1.	Blueberry Muffins	171
2.	Fig Almond Olive Cake	173
3.	Carrot pudding	175
4.	Musicians Dessert	177
5.	Almond Dessert	179
6.	Ice Cream Sandwich Dessert	181
7.	Cold Kiwi Cream Dessert	183
8.	Strawberry Mousse	185
9.	Gluten-Free Raspberry Icebox Pies in a Jar	187
10.	Berry and Cashew Cream Dessert Pizza	189

FRUIT SALADS

1.	Mimosa Fruit Salad	191
2.	Low Fat Fruit Salad	193
3.	Healthy Fruit Salad with Mint Citrus Dressing	195
4.	Paleo Fruit Salad	197
5.	Grilled Fruit Salad with Coconut Cream	199

PASTA, BREAD, RICE

1.	Burritos	201
2.	Light Bread	203
3.	Quesadillas	205
4.	Diet Pasta	207
5.	Easy Brown Rice	209

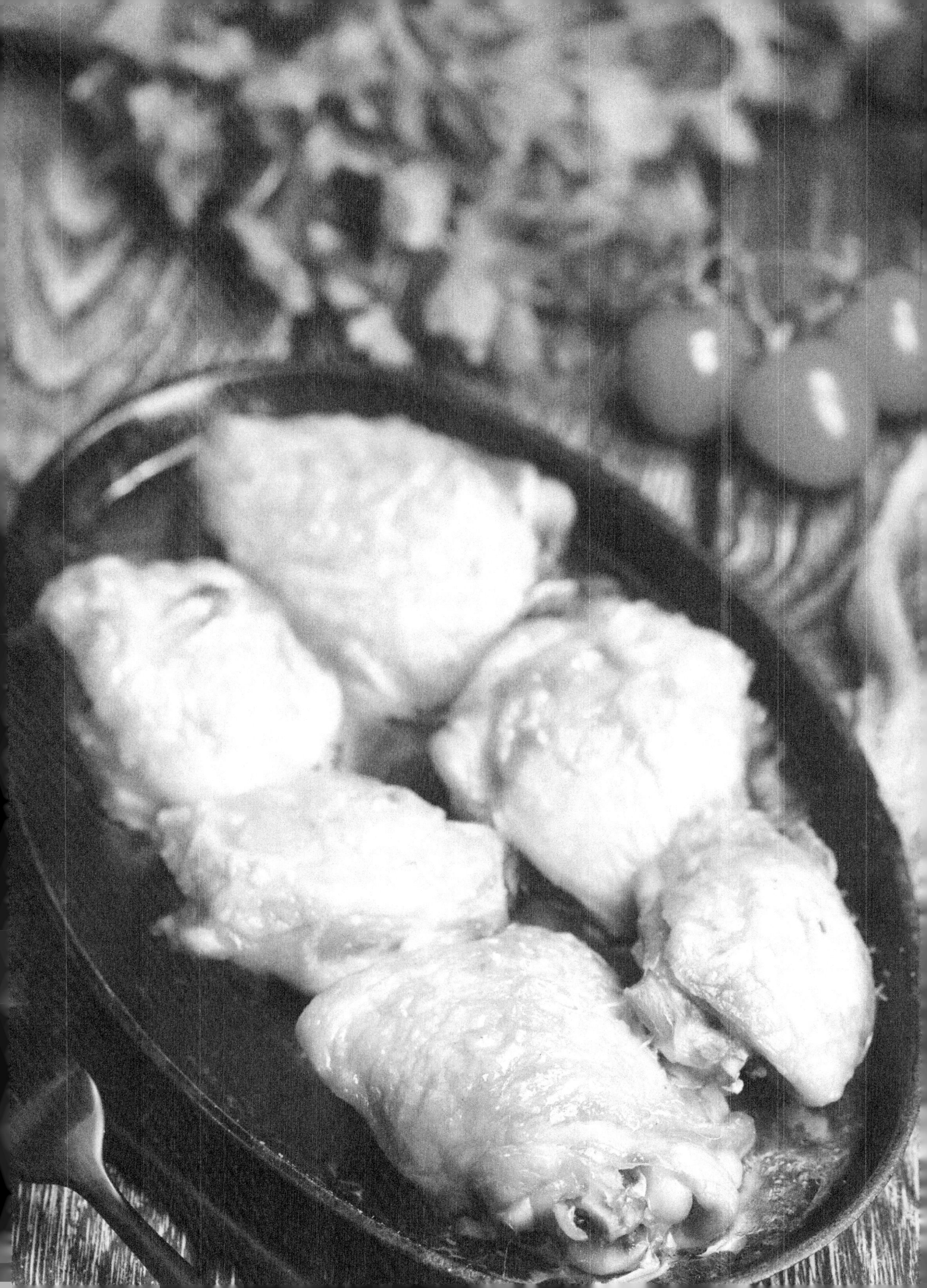

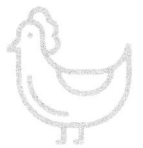

CHIMICHURRI CHICKEN TRAY BAKE

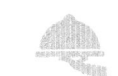
SERVINGS - 4

TIME - 40 mins

 NUTRITIONAL VALUE

- Calories- 643
- Carbohydrates- 7.4g
- Proteins-30.1 g
- Fats-54g

 INGREDIENTS

- 4 chicken thighs
- 1 tsp onion powder
- ½ tsp garlic powder
- ½ cup asparagus
- ½ cup green beans
- ½ cup broccoli florets

Chimichurri sauce
- 1 cup parsley
- 5 garlic cloves
- ¼ cup fresh oregano
- ½ cup olive oil
- 2 tbsp apple cider vinegar
- Salt as per taste
- Black pepper as per taste

 INSTRUCTIONS

1. Preheat your oven to 392 degree Fahrenheit (200 degrees Celsius).
2. Apply all the seasonings to your chicken thighs as set them aside. Put chicken thighs onto a greased baking tray and cook it for 20 minutes.
3. After 20 minutes take out the baking tray and spread greens over the chicken thighs.
4. Cover your baking tray with aluminum foil and bake it for another 10 minutes.
5. To make the chimichurri sauce, take a food processor and add garlic along with all the given ingredients.
6. Serve your chicken thighs along with some chimichurri sauce and enjoy!

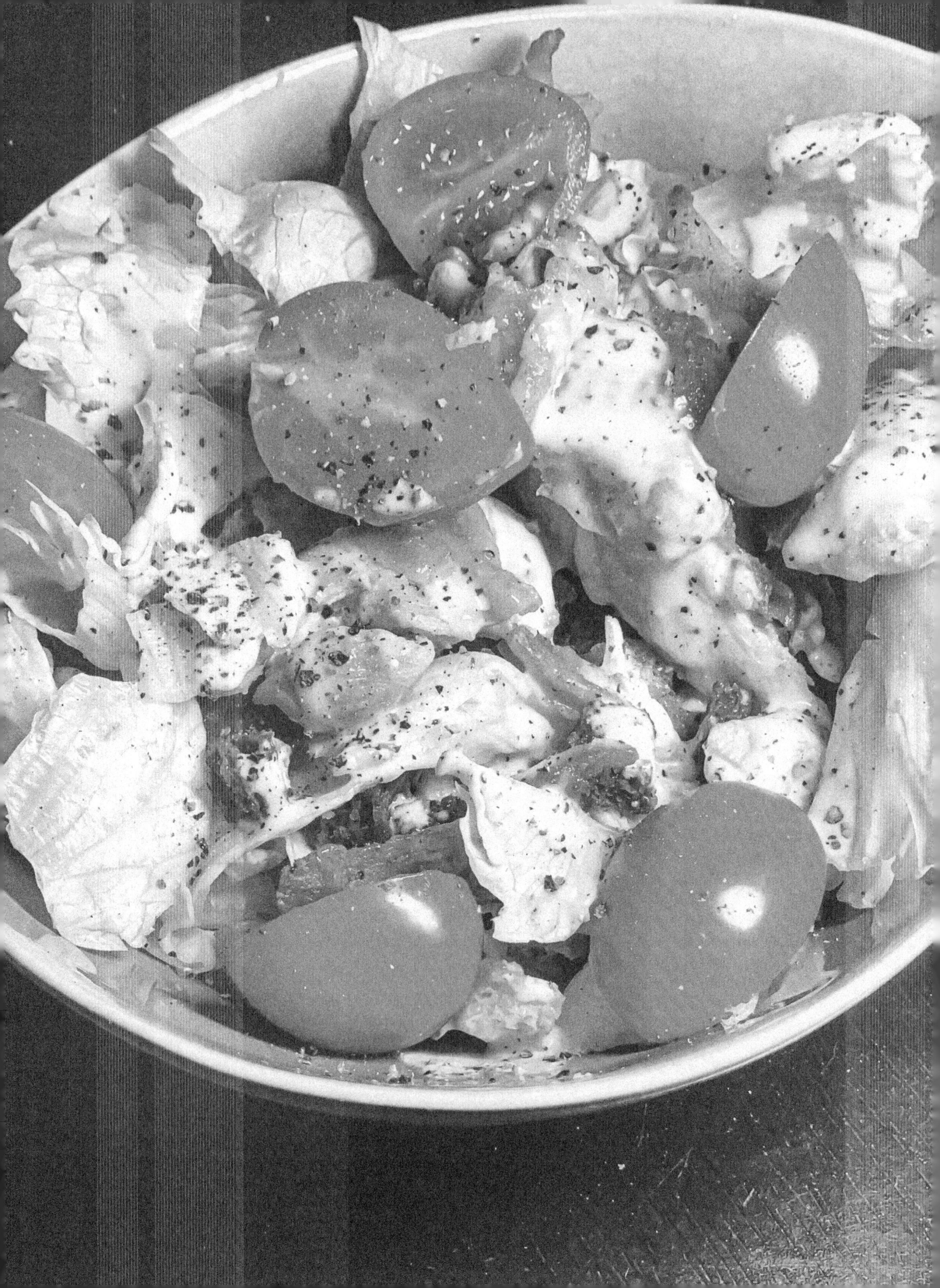

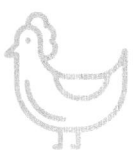# CAPRESE CHICKEN BOWL

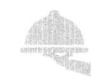
SERVINGS - 1

TIME - 12 hr 30 min

NUTRITIONAL VALUE

- Calories-712 kcal
- Carbohydrates-7.3g
- Proteins-43.5g
- Fats-54.2g

INGREDIENTS

INSTRUCTIONS

Marinating Chicken
- 1 chicken breast
- 1 tbsp olive oil
- 1 tsp vinegar
- 1 tsp Italian seasoning
- Salt as per taste

Salad
- 2 cups spinach leaves
- ¼ cup basil leaves
- ¼ cup mozzarella balls
- ¼ cup sliced avocado
- 1/3 cup halved cherry tomatoes

Dressing
- 1 tbsp olive oil
- 1 tsp vinegar
- Salt as per taste
- Black pepper as per taste

1. Marinade chicken with the required ingredients and place them in the refrigerator for 12 hours.
2. Next heat a grill pan and grill the chicken breast on both sides until it's cooked and is tender.
3. Next, prepare the dressing by mixing all the ingredients.
4. Prepare your salad portion by combing all the veggies and cheese balls together.
5. Serve the diet portion by making a plate and assembling chicken breast, salad along with some dressing on top.

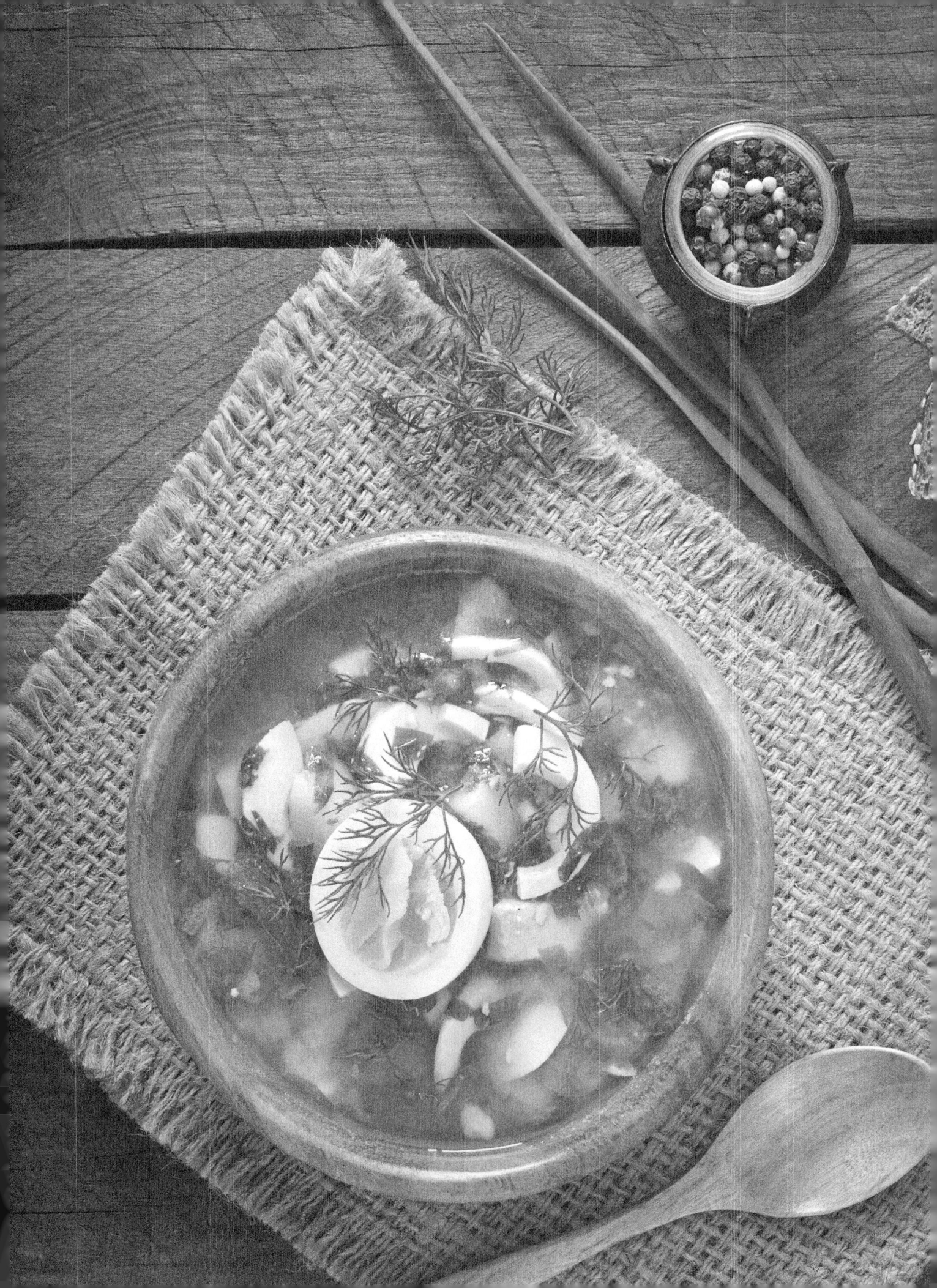

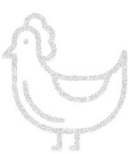

CHICKEN AND SPINACH SOUP

SERVINGS - 5

TIME - 30 min

 NUTRITIONAL VALUE

- Calories-227kcal
- Carbohydrates-18g
- Proteins-20g
- Fats-10g

 INGREDIENTS

 **INSTRUCTIONS**

- 3 tbsp extra virgin olive oil
- ½ cup carrot
- 1 chicken breasts
- 1 large minced garlic clove
- 5 cups chicken broth
- 1 ½ tsp dried marjoram
- 1 cup baby spinach
- 1 can cannellini beans
- ¼ cup grated parmesan
- 1/3 cup basil leaves
- Black pepper as per taste
- ¾ cup plain yogurt

1. Heat a saucepan with 2 tbsp olive oil and add carrots plus chicken into it. Fry them until the color of the chicken changes.
2. Add some garlic and cook for another 1 min. Then add broth marjoram and bring the contents of the pan to a boil.
3. Simmer the contents for 5 minutes.
4. Remove chicken pieces from the broth and transfer them to a cutting board. Add spinach pieces and beans to the broth and cook for 10 minutes.
5. Add olive oil, parmesan, and basil to a food processor. Spin the processor until a smooth consistency is obtained.
6. Add chicken pieces and paste into the bowl and season your soup with salt and pepper.

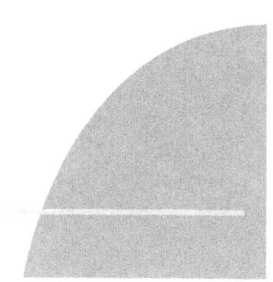

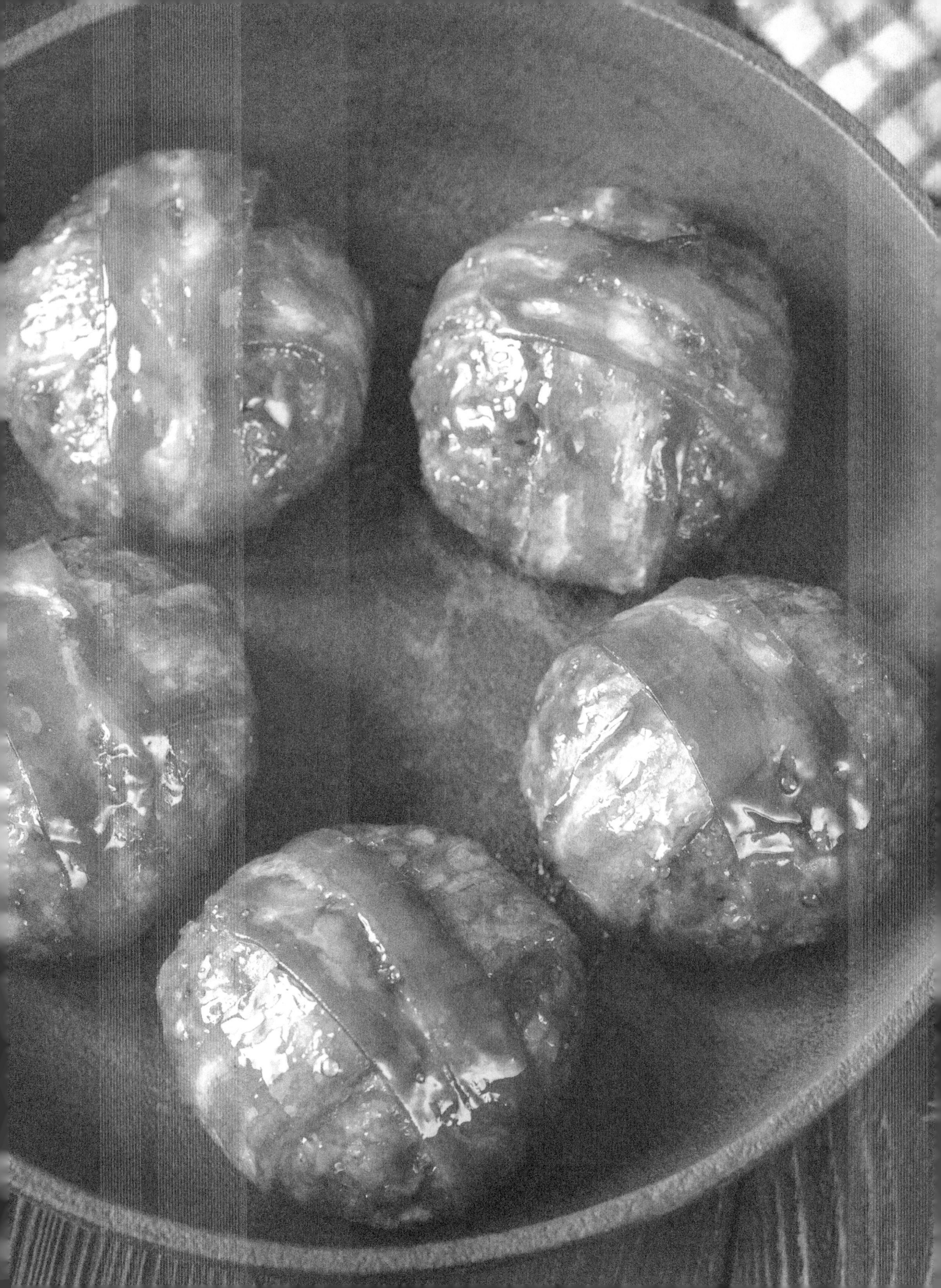

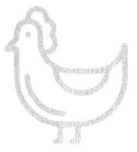
BACON-WRAPPED CHICKEN PARCELS

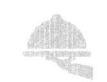
SERVINGS - 4

TIME - 30 min

NUTRITIONAL VALUE

- Calories-492 kcal
- Carbohydrates-2.1g
- Proteins-57.6g
- Fats-29.5g

INGREDIENTS

- 4 medium chicken breasts
- 1 cup cream cheese
- ½ cup parmesan cheese
- 2 tbsp chopped parsley
- Salt as per taste
- 8 thin slices of bacon

INSTRUCTIONS

1. Prepare the cheese stuffing by mixing cream cheese, parmesan, and parsley into a bowl. Divide the mixture into 4 portions and with the help of a cling roll them into long logs. Freeze these cheese cylinders.
2. Prepare the chicken by making pockets into the chicken breast pieces. Stuff in frozen cheese logs and wrap them with bacon slices.
3. Pre-heat your oven at 400 degrees Fahrenheit (200 degrees Celsius) and cook your chicken breast pieces for 25 minutes.
4. Serve with any dip.

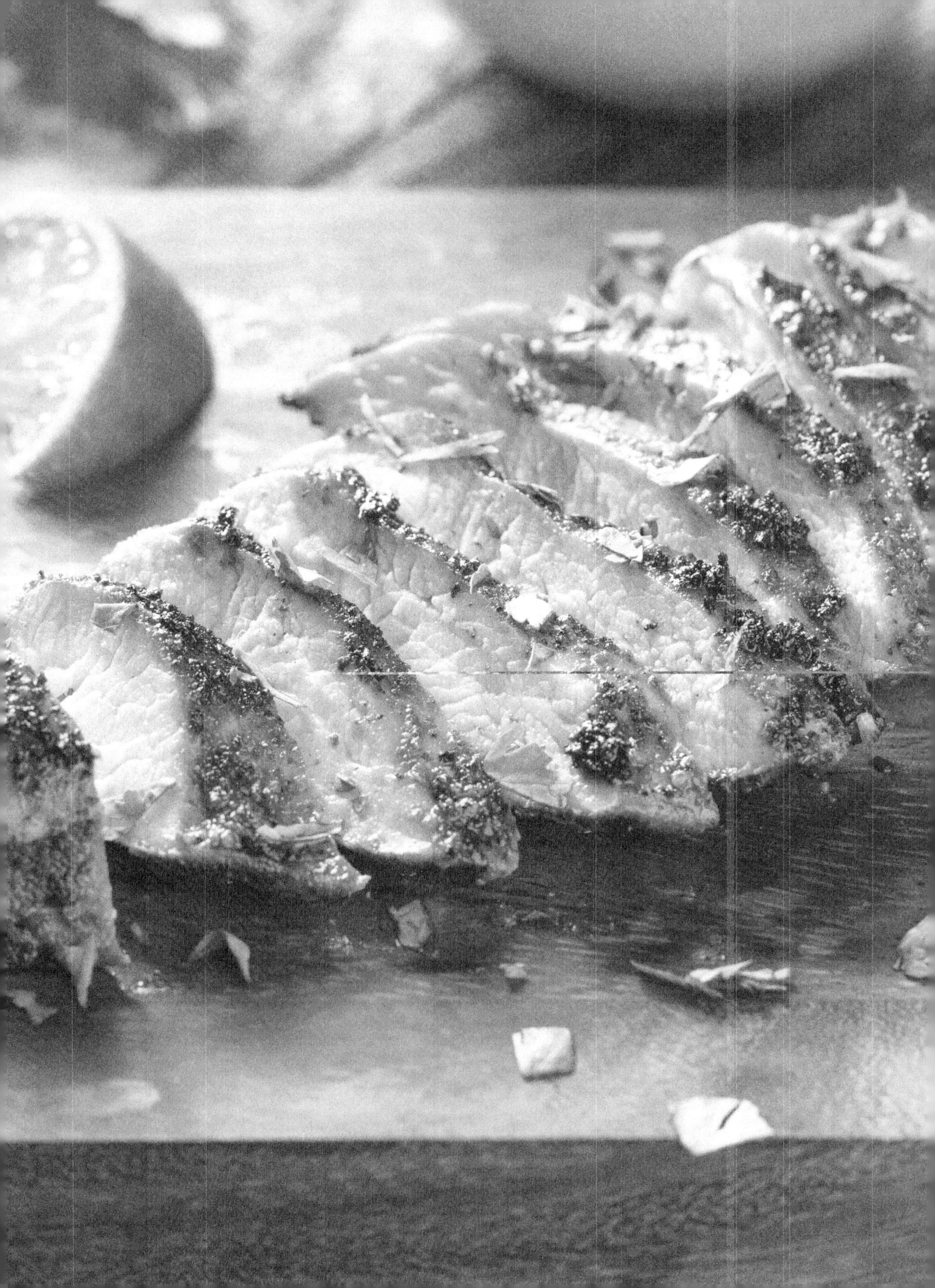

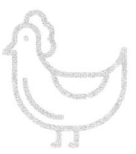
CHIPOTLE CHICKEN

SERVINGS - 2

TIME - 30 min

 NUTRITIONAL VALUE

- Calories- 817 cal
- Carbohydrates-20.9g
- Proteins-57.9g
- Fats-58.9g

 INGREDIENTS

- 4 slices bacon
- 2 chicken breasts
- 1 sliced avocado
- ¼ sliced onion
- 1 small sliced tomatoes
- 2 leaves of lettuce
- 2 cheese slices
- 2 freshly made wheat buns
- 2 tbsp mayonnaise
- 1 tbsp minced chipotle
- 1 tbsp adobo sauce

 INSTRUCTIONS

1. To prepare chipotle mayonnaise mix mayonnaise, chipotle, and adobo together. Set it aside.
2. Fry the bacon until crispy and set it aside.
3. Season the chicken breast pieces with salt and pepper. Grill them onto the same pan that was used to fry bacon slices for 5 minutes on each side.
4. Toast buns on the same pan and assemble all the ingredients to make a perfect burger for your healthy lifestyle.

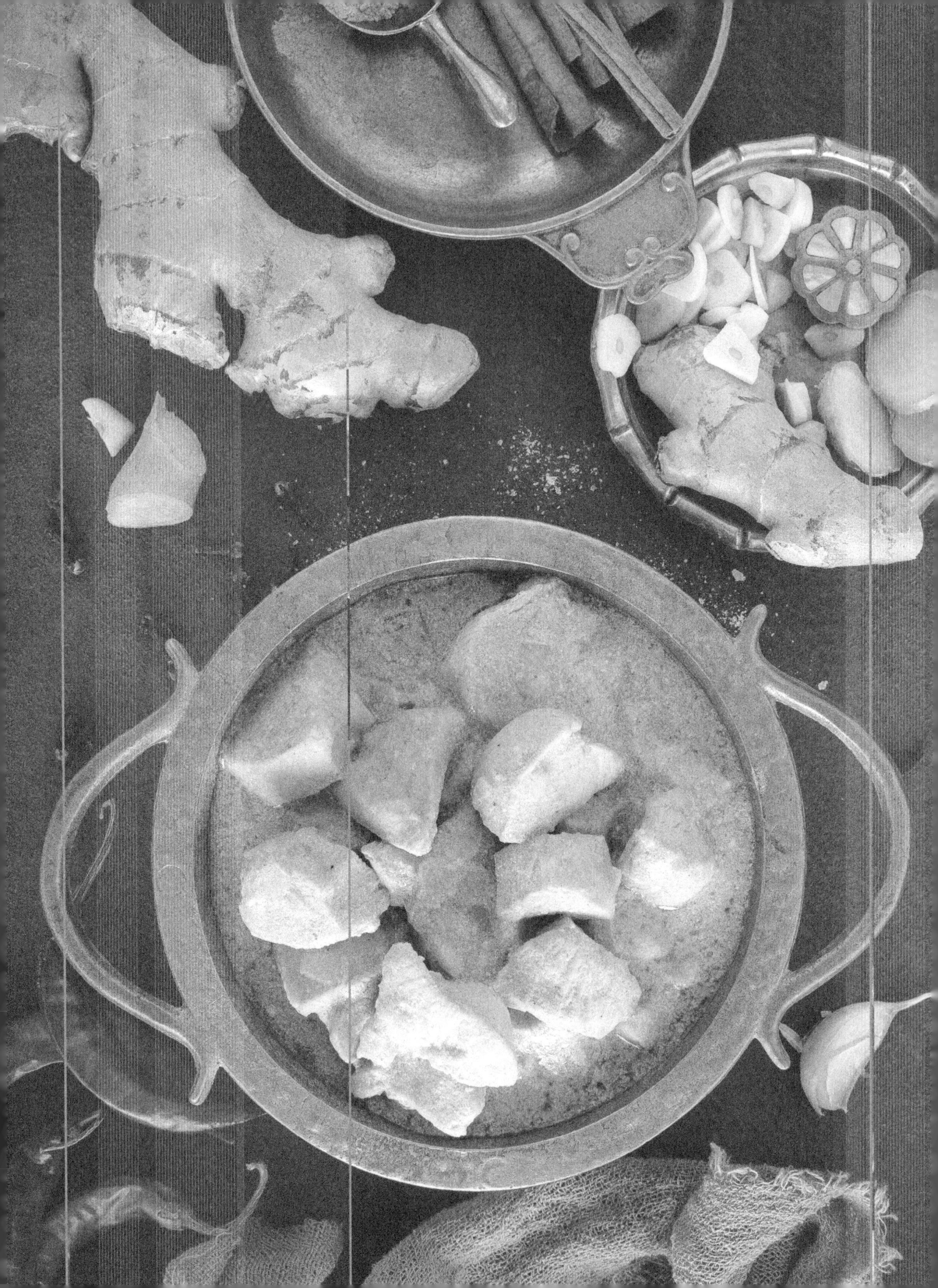

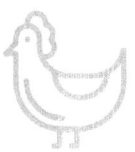# COCONUT CHICKEN CURRY

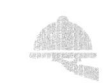
SERVINGS - 4

TIME - 40 min

 NUTRITIONAL VALUE

- Calories-503 Kcal
- Carbohydrates-11.4g
- Proteins-34.7g
- Fats-35g

 INGREDIENTS

- 2 cups chicken filet
- 1 ½ cup coconut milk
- 1 cup chopped bell red pepper
- ½ cup broccoli
- 1 diced small onion
- 1 diced small carrot
- 1 tbsp chopped ginger
- 1 minced garlic clove
- A handful of cashews

Seasonings
- 1 tbsp red curry paste
- 1 tsp coriander powder
- 1 tbsp curry powder
- Salt as per taste
- Black pepper as per taste

 INSTRUCTIONS

1. In a skillet heat a bit of oil and add onions, garlic, and ginger into it. Sauté it for minutes.
2. Add chicken pieces into the same skillet and cook for 10 minutes. Also, add some curry paste to the chicken pieces and cook for 2 minutes.
3. Now add coconut milk and cook.
4. Also, add some bell pepper and broccoli into the pot.
5. Season with a spice mix and salt and pepper.
6. Reduce the heat and cook the curry on low flame for 15 minutes.

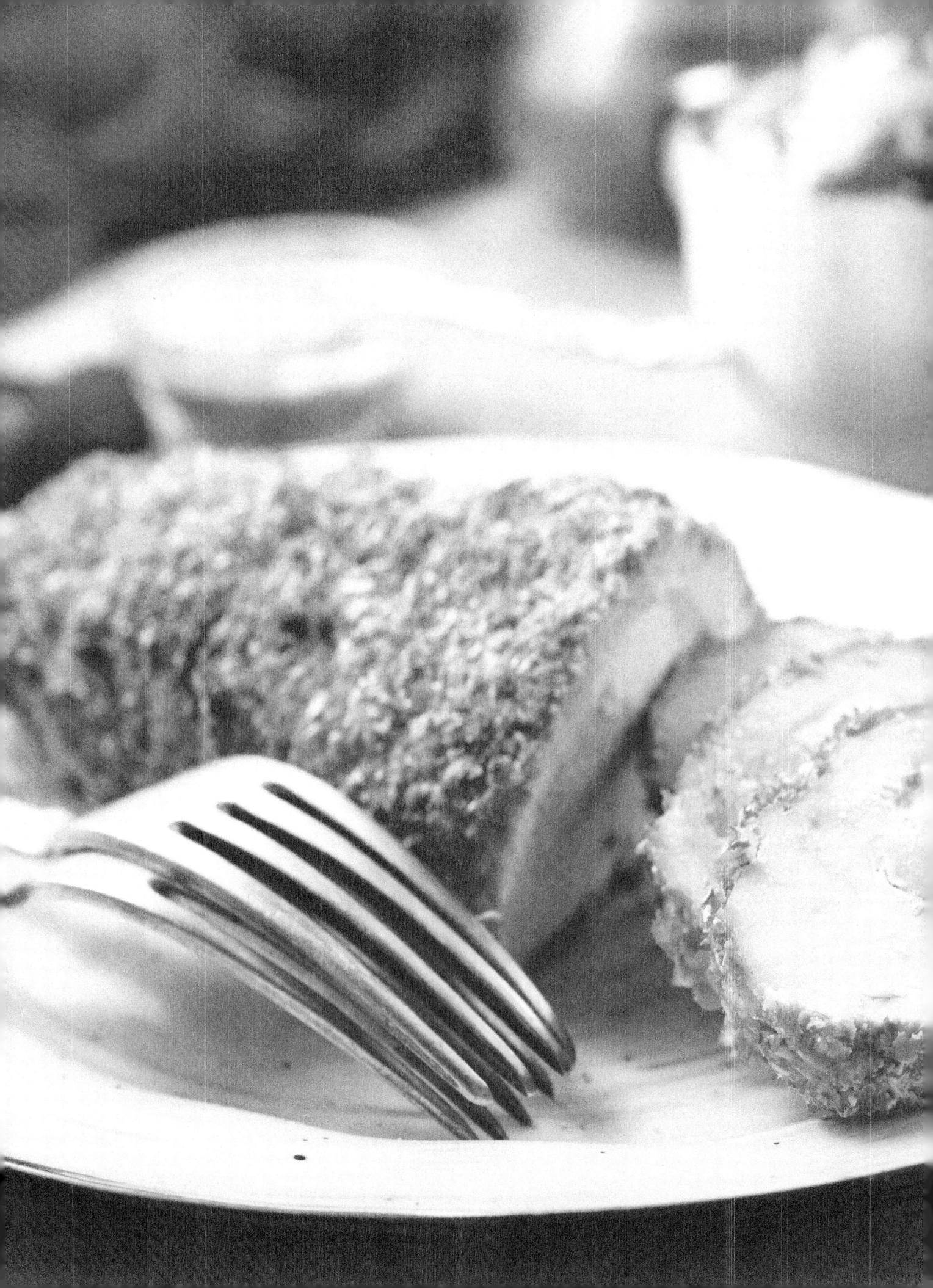

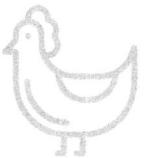

PAILLARD OF CHICKEN WITH LEMON AND HERBS

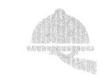

SERVINGS - 6

TIME - 25 min

 NUTRITIONAL VALUE

- Calories-240 k cal
- Carbohydrates-1g
- Proteins-32g
- Fats-12g

 INGREDIENTS

- 6 chicken breasts
- 2 tbsp olive oil
- ½ tbsp. vinegar
- ½ cup parmesan
- 2 minced garlic cloves
- 3 chopped rosemary
- 6 shredded sage leaves
- ½ tbsp lemon juice
- 3 tbsp olive oil

 INSTRUCTIONS

1. With the help of a meat basher, bash chicken breast pieces to make them in the form of thin layers.
2. Marinade chicken pieces by adding shredded garlic cloves, rosemary, sage, and mix everything well. Also add lemon juice, olive oil, and some black pepper. Marinade chicken pieces for at least 2 hours.
3. Cook chicken pieces onto a grill on both sides until they are golden brown.
4. In a bowl add oil and vinegar. Also, add some seasoning and parmesan cheese. Serve it with chicken pieces.

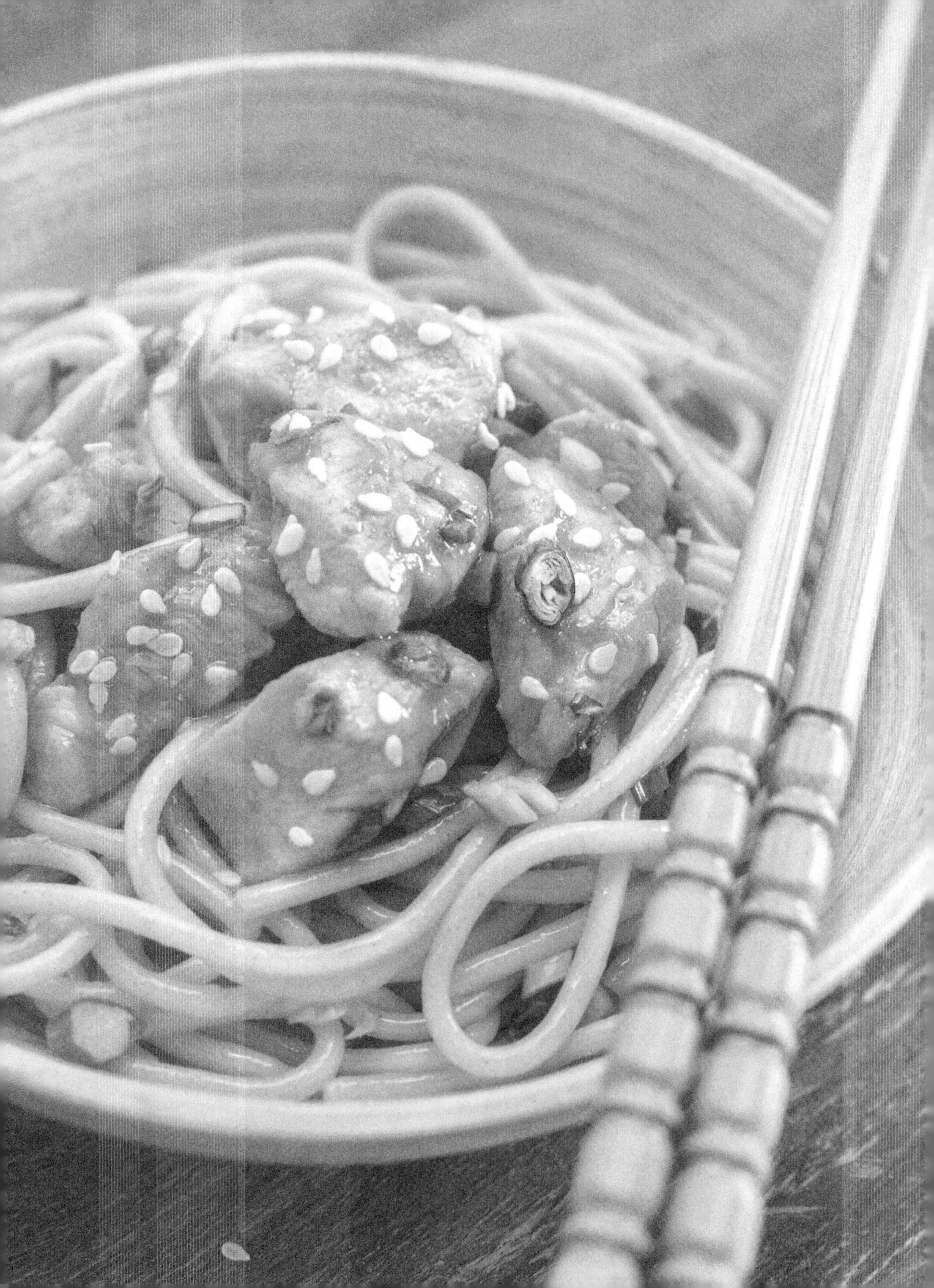

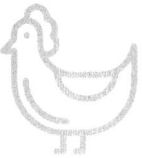

LEMON PARMESAN CHICKEN WITH ZUCCHINI NOODLES

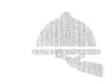

SERVINGS - 4

TIME - 30 min

NUTRITIONAL VALUE

- Calories-412 k cal
- Carbohydrates-6.3g
- Proteins-88.3g
- Fats-17.8g

INGREDIENTS

- 4 zucchini spirals
- ½ kg boneless chicken
- 1 tsp rock salt
- ½ tsp ground black pepper
- 2 tsp olive oil
- 4 minced garlic cloves
- 2 tsp dried oregano
- 2 tbsp butter
- 2 tsp lemon zest
- 2 tbsp parsley
- 1 sliced lemon
- 2/3 cup vegetable broth
- 1/3 cup parmesan

INSTRUCTIONS

1. Blanch zucchini spirals to form zucchini noodles
2. Apply salt and pepper to chicken pieces and marinate them for 10 minutes.
3. In a large skillet add olive oil and cook chicken pieces until nice crisp golden brown color appears.
4. To the same skillet add garlic and sauté it for 1 minute. Now add butter, lemon zest, and oregano.
5. Add vegetable broth to the pan and cook until bubbles are formed.
6. Add parmesan cheese to the soup mixture along with some chicken pieces.
7. Garnish zucchini noodles with lemon slices and parsley and serve them with soup.

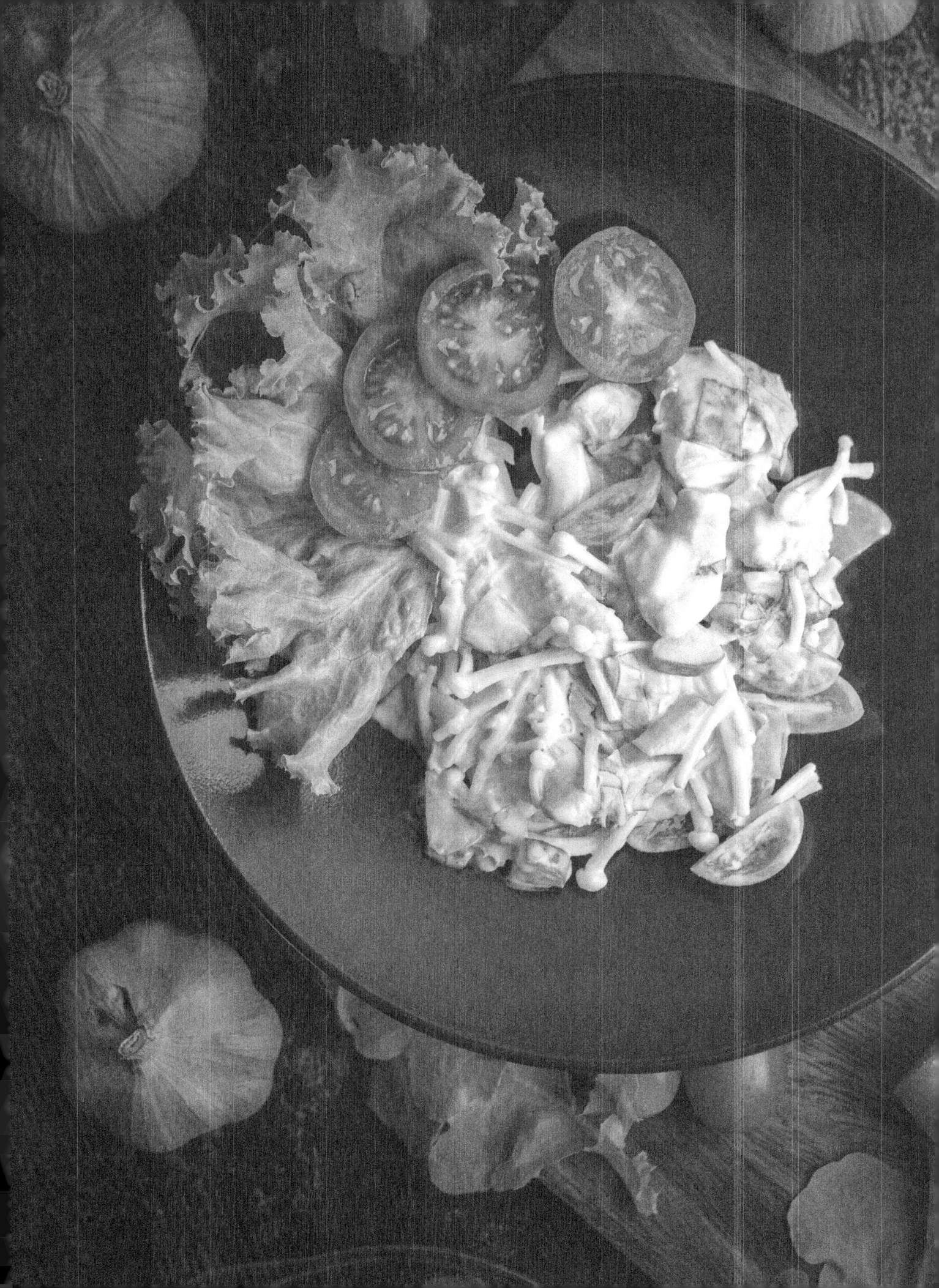

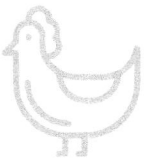

CREAMY PESTO CHICKEN SALAD WITH GREENS

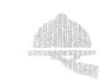

SERVINGS - 3

TIME - 15 min

NUTRITIONAL VALUE

- Calories- 419 kcal
- Carbohydrates-7.8g
- Proteins-35.4g
- Fats-28g

INGREDIENTS

- 1 pound boneless chicken
- ¼ cup pesto
- ¼ cup low-fat mayonnaise
- 3 tbsp chopped red onion
- 2 tbsp olive oil
- 2 tbsp vinegar
- ¼ tsp salt
- ¼ tsp ground black pepper
- 2 cups mixed salad greens
- 1 cup halved cherry tomatoes

INSTRUCTIONS

1. Boil chicken pieces and shred them.
2. In a mixing bowl add in some mayonnaise, pesto, red onion, and vinegar and mix them.
3. Add shredded chicken pieces into the same mixing bowl along with some olive oil, salt, black pepper, mixed greens, and cherry tomatoes.
4. Mix everything gently and serve!

OMAD DIET BOOK

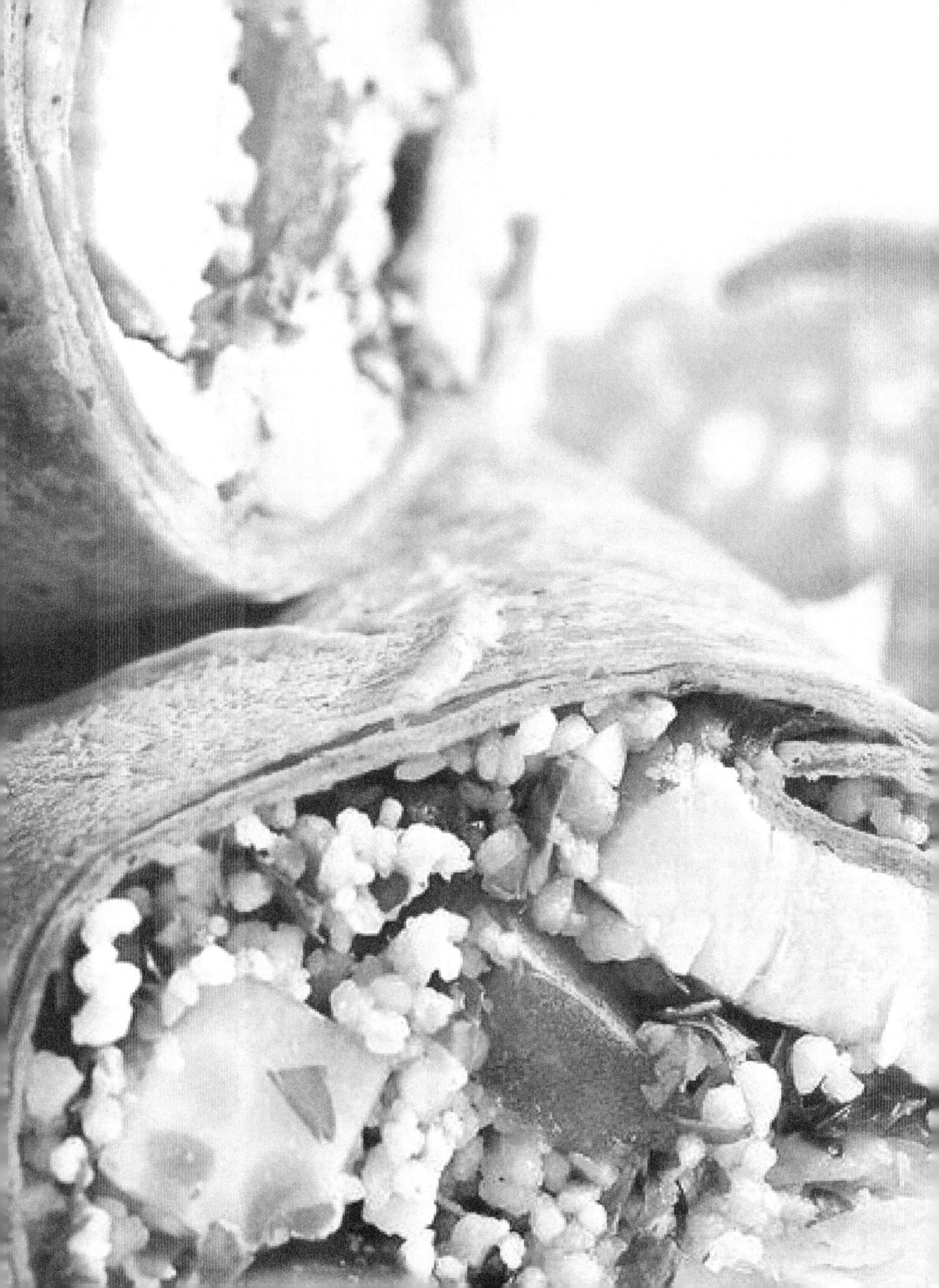

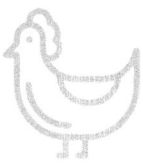

CHICKEN AND APPLE KALE WRAPS

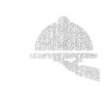

SERVINGS - 3

TIME - 5 min

NUTRITIONAL VALUE

- Calories-251 kcal
- Carbohydrates-22g
- Proteins-31g
- Fats-7g

INGREDIENTS

- 1 tbsp mayonnaise
- 1 tsp mustard
- 3 kale leaves
- 3 slices of cooked chicken
- 6 pieces of red onion
- 1 sliced apple

INSTRUCTIONS

1. In a mixing bowl add mayonnaise and mustard to form a paste.
2. Apply a fine layer of this paste onto the kale leaves and place pieces of chicken, onions, and apple in the center of the leaves.
3. Finally, wrap up the kale leaves to prepare kale wraps.

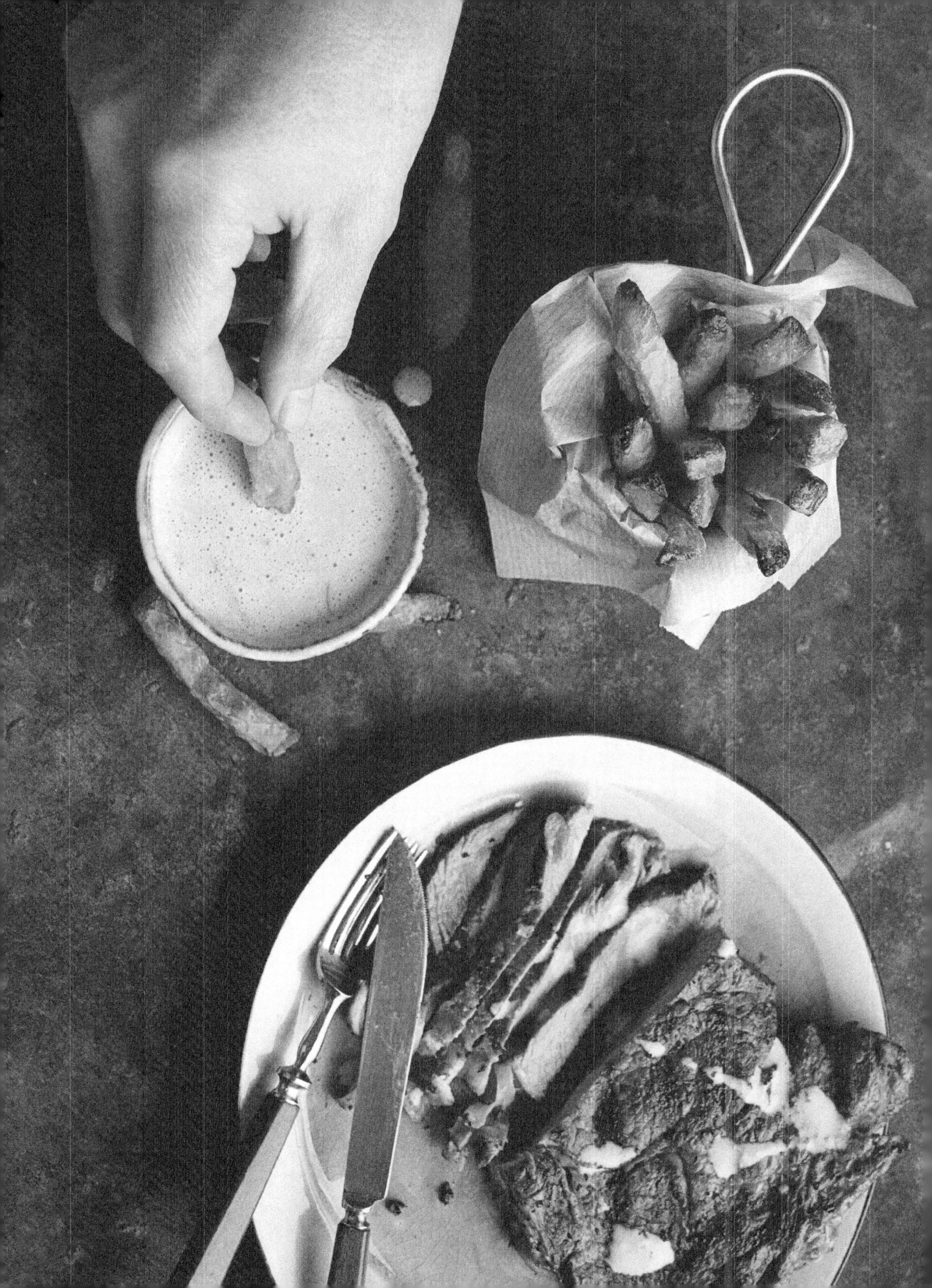

STEAK DINNER FOR TWO

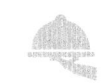

SERVINGS - 2

TIME - 30 min

NUTRITIONAL VALUE

- Calories- 1221 kcal
- Proteins – 56.7 g
- Carbohydrates-4.4 g
- Fats- 107.8 g

INGREDIENTS

INSTRUCTIONS

Hollandaise Sauce
- ½ cup extra virgin olive oil
- 3 egg yolks
- 2 tbsp lemon juice
- 2 tbsp chopped dried tomatoes
- 1 tbsp chopped basil
- Salt to taste
- Pepper to taste

Steak
- 2 beefsteaks
- 1 tsp olive oil
- Salt as per taste
- Pepper as per taste

Grilled Asparagus
- 14 asparagus spears
- 1 tbsp extra virgin olive oil
- Salt as per taste
- Pepper as per taste

1. To prepare hollandaise sauce, take a jar and add olive oil, egg yolk, lemon juice, salt, chopped dried tomatoes, basil, and pepper into the jar of a hand blender. Blend all the ingredients until a sauce-like consistency is obtained.
2. To prepare steak, heat your grill pan to the point and season it with salt and pepper. Also, apply some olive oil to the steak.
3. Grill steaks on the pan. on the pan.
4. Take asparagus and apply some olive oil, salt, and pepper to it. Grill them also on the same pan and serve everything together.

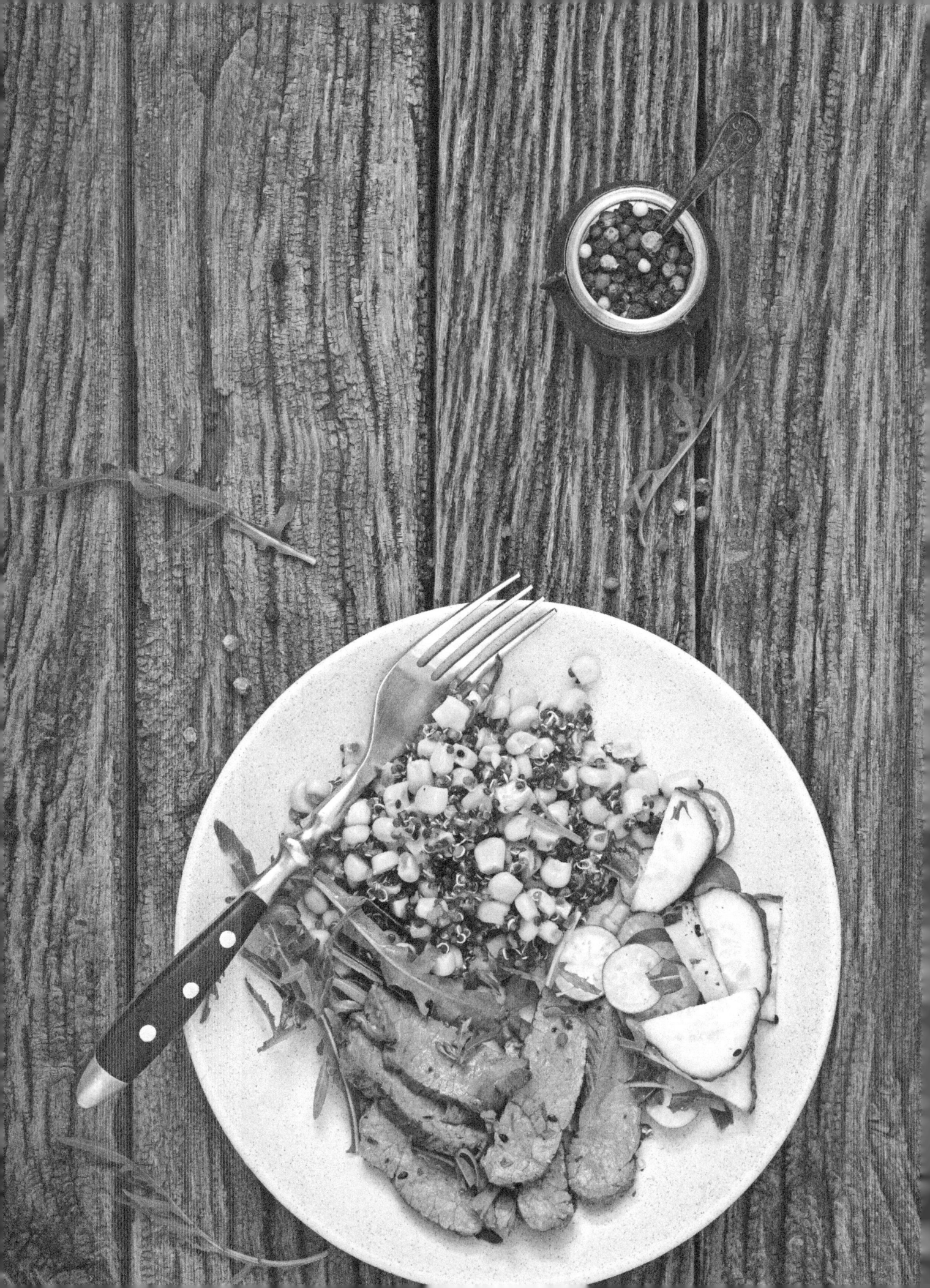

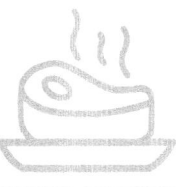

STEAK TACO BOWL

SERVINGS - 1

TIME - 20 min

 NUTRITIONAL VALUE

- Calories-702 kcal
- Carbohydrates-8.8g
- Proteins-34.3g
- Fats-56.1g

 INGREDIENTS

 INSTRUCTIONS

Steak Bowl
- 1 cup beef steak
- 1 tbsp oil
- Salt as per taste
- Black pepper as per taste
- 1 cup cooked cauliflower rice
- 2 tbsp minced cilantro
- 1 tsp lime juice

Toppings
- ½ sliced avocado
- ¼ cup salsa
- 1 tbsp sour cream
- ½ sliced jalapeno pepper
- 2 sliced radish

1. Season your steak with salt and pepper and grill them onto a grilling pan. Grill steak for 5 minutes on both sides and set it aside. Cut it into smaller pieces.
2. Assemble your bowl by adding lemon juice and cilantro into the cauliflower rice.
3. Top up your bowl with toppings and serve.

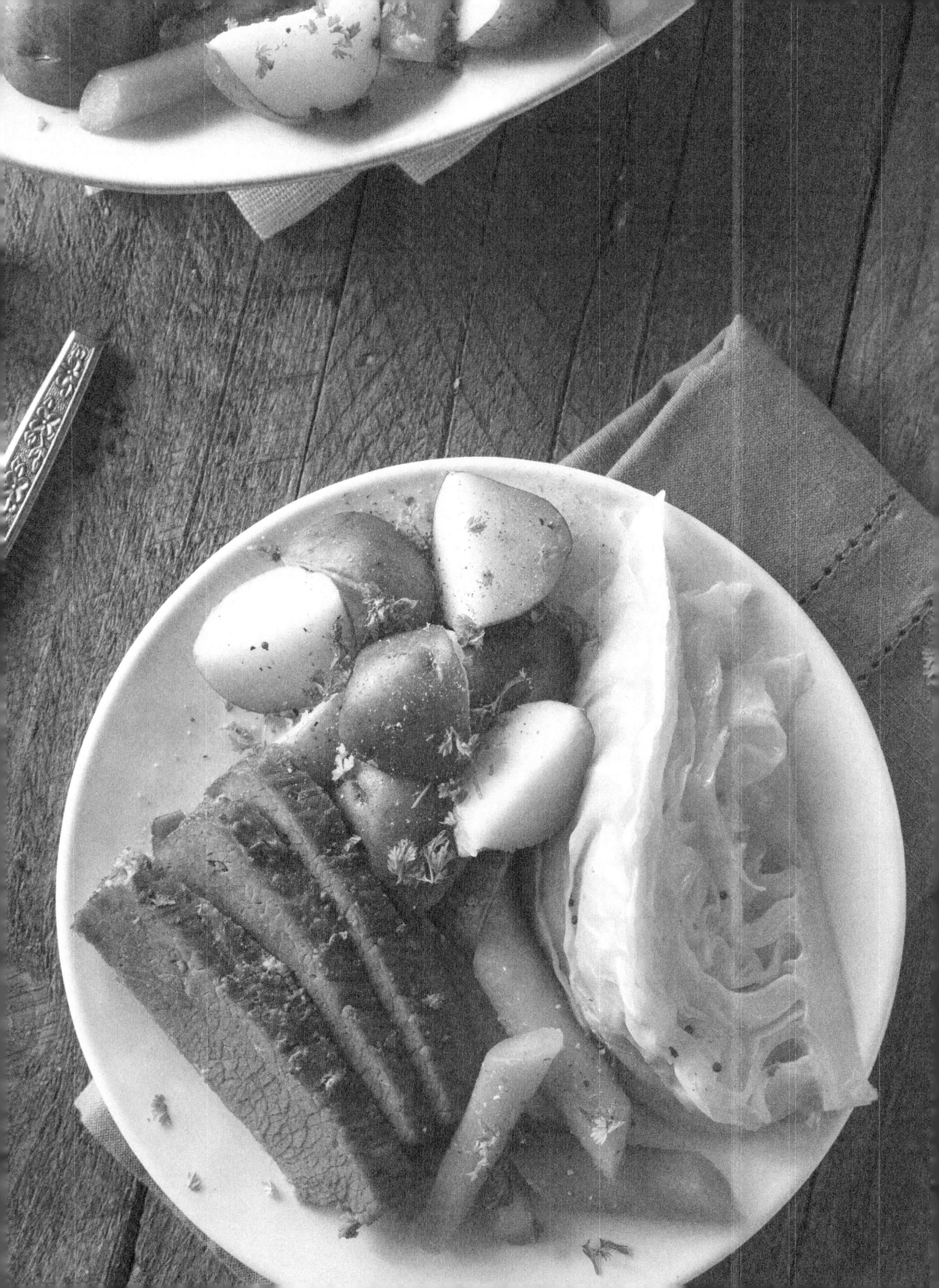

CORNED BEEF AND CABBAGE

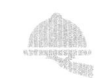

SERVINGS - 6

TIME - 4 Hrs

 NUTRITIONAL VALUE

- Calories- 312 cal
- Carbohydrates-26.9g
- Proteins-14.8g
- Fats-14.4g

 INGREDIENTS

- 3 cups corned beef
- 2 diced onions
- 4 celery stalks
- 1 tbsp pickling spices
- Salt as per taste
- Black pepper as per taste
- 1 green cabbage
- 2 carrots
- ½ cup mustard
- 2 tbsp apple cider vinegar
- ¼ cup mayonnaise
- 2 tbsp roughly chopped capers
- 1 tsp capers brine
- 2 tbsp chopped parsley

 INSTRUCTIONS

1. Take a deep pot and add corned beef, onion, celery, and pickling spices into it. Add water into the pot and cook it till a boil comes in it. Simmer the contents for 2 hours until the beef becomes tender.
2. Add cabbage and carrots and continue to simmer the pot contents for another 45 minutes.
3. Remove the veggies from the pot and slice the corned beef into normal slices.
4. In a small bowl whisk mustard, vinegar and season it with salt and pepper.
5. In another mix mayonnaise, capers, brine, and parsley. Season it with salt and pepper.
6. Serve corned beef slices with both sauces and enjoy!

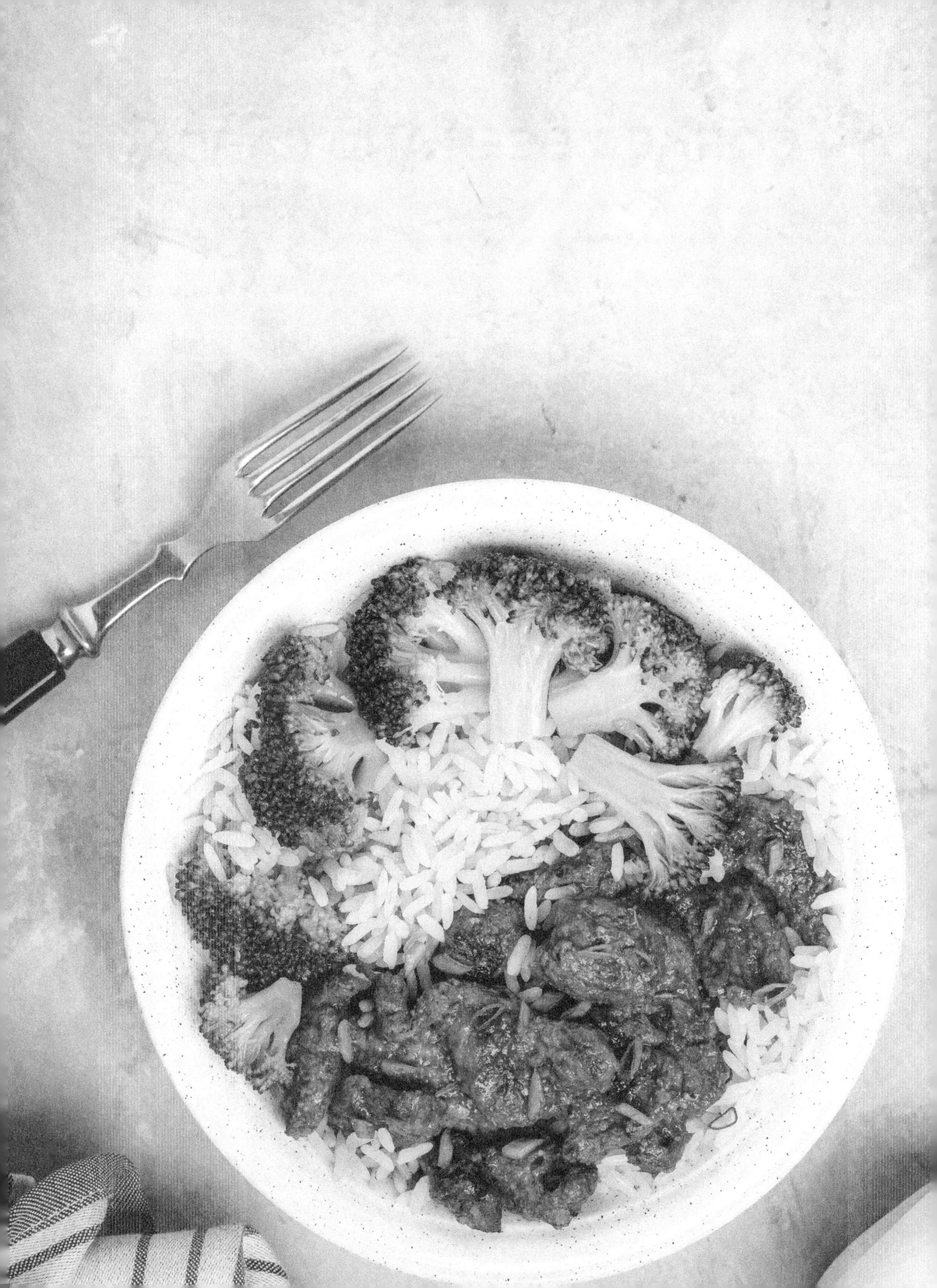

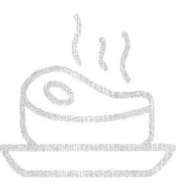

GROUND BEEF AND BROCCOLI

SERVINGS - 4

TIME - 30 min

 NUTRITIONAL VALUE

- Calories-699 k cal
- Carbohydrates-3.7g
- Proteins-77.2g
- Fats-42g

 INGREDIENTS

- 2 cups ground beef
- ¼ cup olive oil
- 1 cup broccoli
- 1 tsp salt
- 1 tsp pepper

 INSTRUCTIONS

1. Take a cooking pan and add oil to it.
2. Add beef along with broccoli and fry until the beef changes its color.
3. Then season the dish with salt and pepper and simmer the contents for 20 minutes.

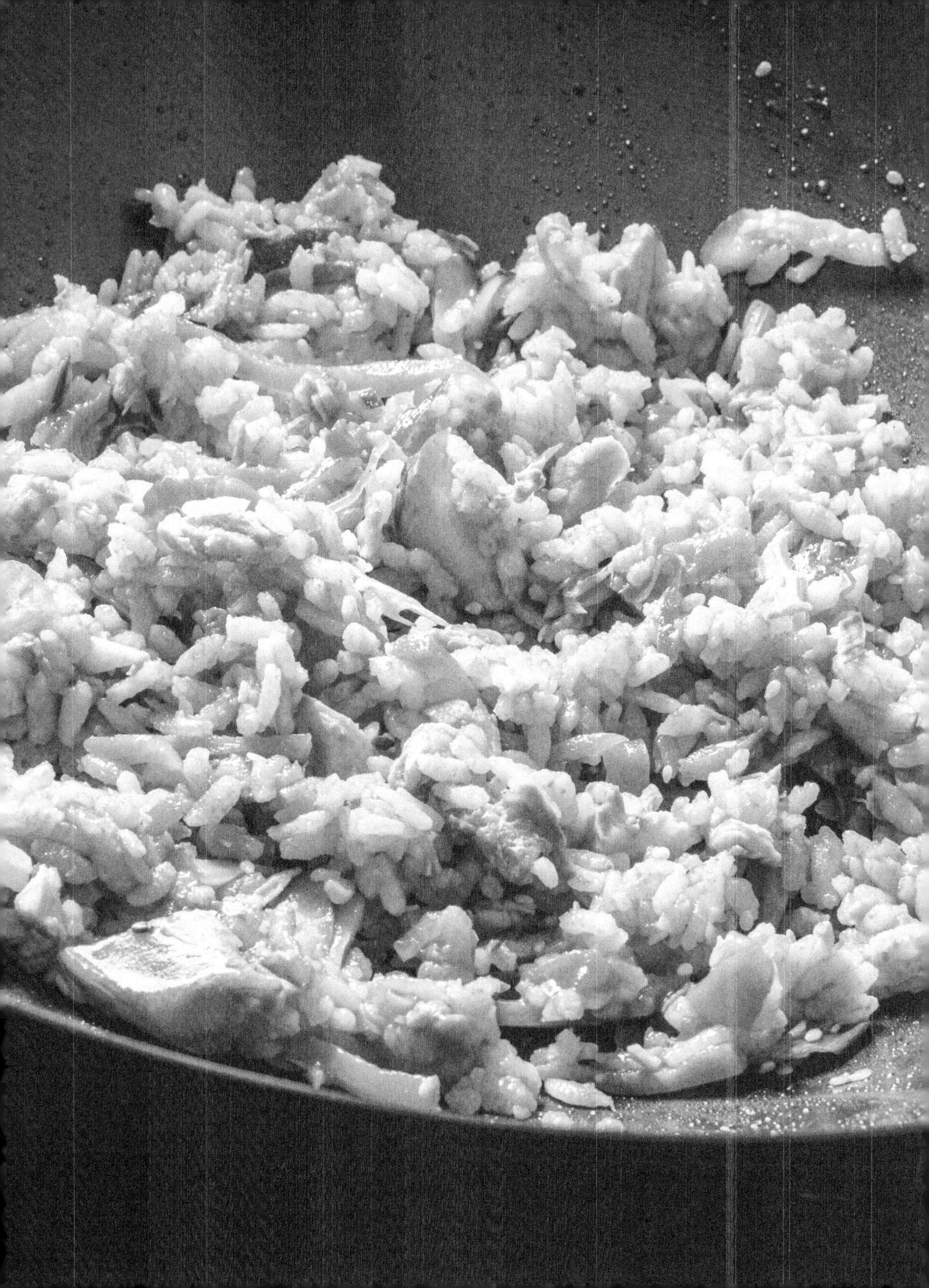

MEDITERRANEAN BEEF AND RICE

SERVINGS - 4

TIME - 40 min

 NUTRITIONAL VALUE

- Calories-255kcal
- Carbohydrates-13g
- Proteins-5g
- Fats-16g

 INGREDIENTS

- 1 ½ cup ground beef
- ½ cup rice
- 1 chopped onion
- 1 minced garlic
- 1 tbsp olive oil
- 1 chopped tomato
- 1 tsp cumin
- 1 tsp coriander
- 1 tsp mint
- 1 tsp paprika
- 1 cup green beans

 INSTRUCTIONS

1. Take a cooking pot and add oil to it. Then add ground beef and fry until the beef releases its juices and add a bit of water to cook it further.
2. Add cumin, coriander, mint, and paprika, and simmer the beef.
3. Also, add some chopped onions and tomatoes along with some garlic.
4. Add rice in it with 1/3 cup of water. Cook while the pot is being covered.
5. Also, add some green beans and tomatoes and stir them in the rice mixture.
6. Serve it hot with a salad of your choice!

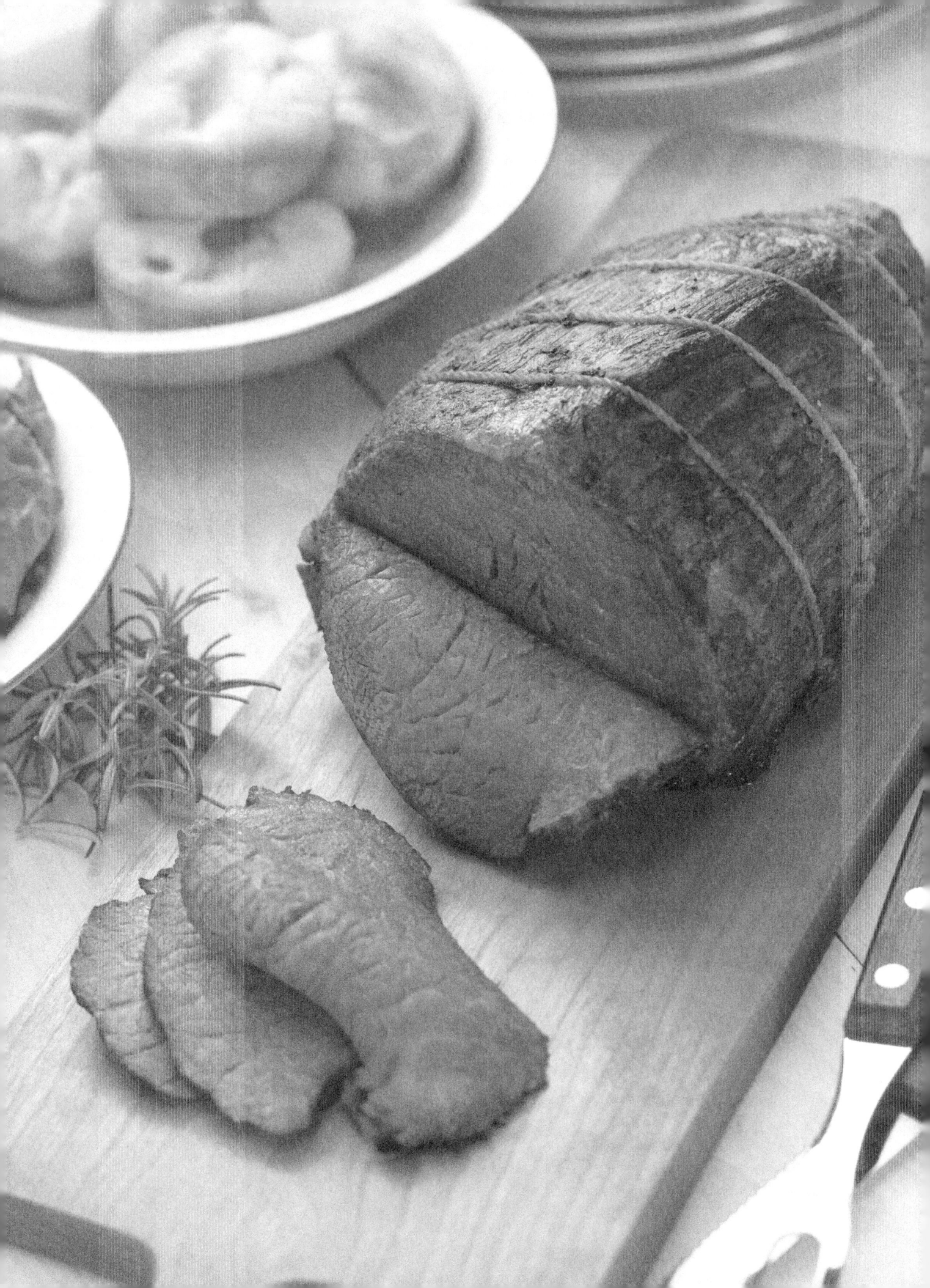

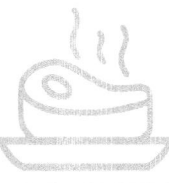

ROASTED BEEF DINNER

SERVINGS - 3

TIME - 5 Hrs

 NUTRITIONAL VALUE

- Calories-414kcal
- Carbohydrates-25g
- Proteins-33g
- Fats-18g

 INGREDIENTS

- 3 cups boneless beef chunks
- 3 cups root vegetables
- 2 onions chopped
- 4 celery stalks
- 2 cup diced tomatoes
- 1 cup chicken broth
- 1 tbsp chopped ginger
- 2 tsp dried oregano
- 1 tsp ground coriander

 INSTRUCTIONS

1. Take a slow cooker pot and add vegetables at the bottom.
2. Layer up beef chunks on top of the vegetables.
3. Add tomatoes and broth along with all the spices in the cooker.
4. Cook it for 4 hours on low flame in the cooker.
5. Take out meat chunks and vegetables. Don't discard the juices.
6. Transfer juices to a saucepan and heat them for 5 min. this is the process of reducing your juice to make a smooth sauce.
7. Prepare your serving plate by adding beef chunks along with some vegetables and a sauce being drizzled on everything.

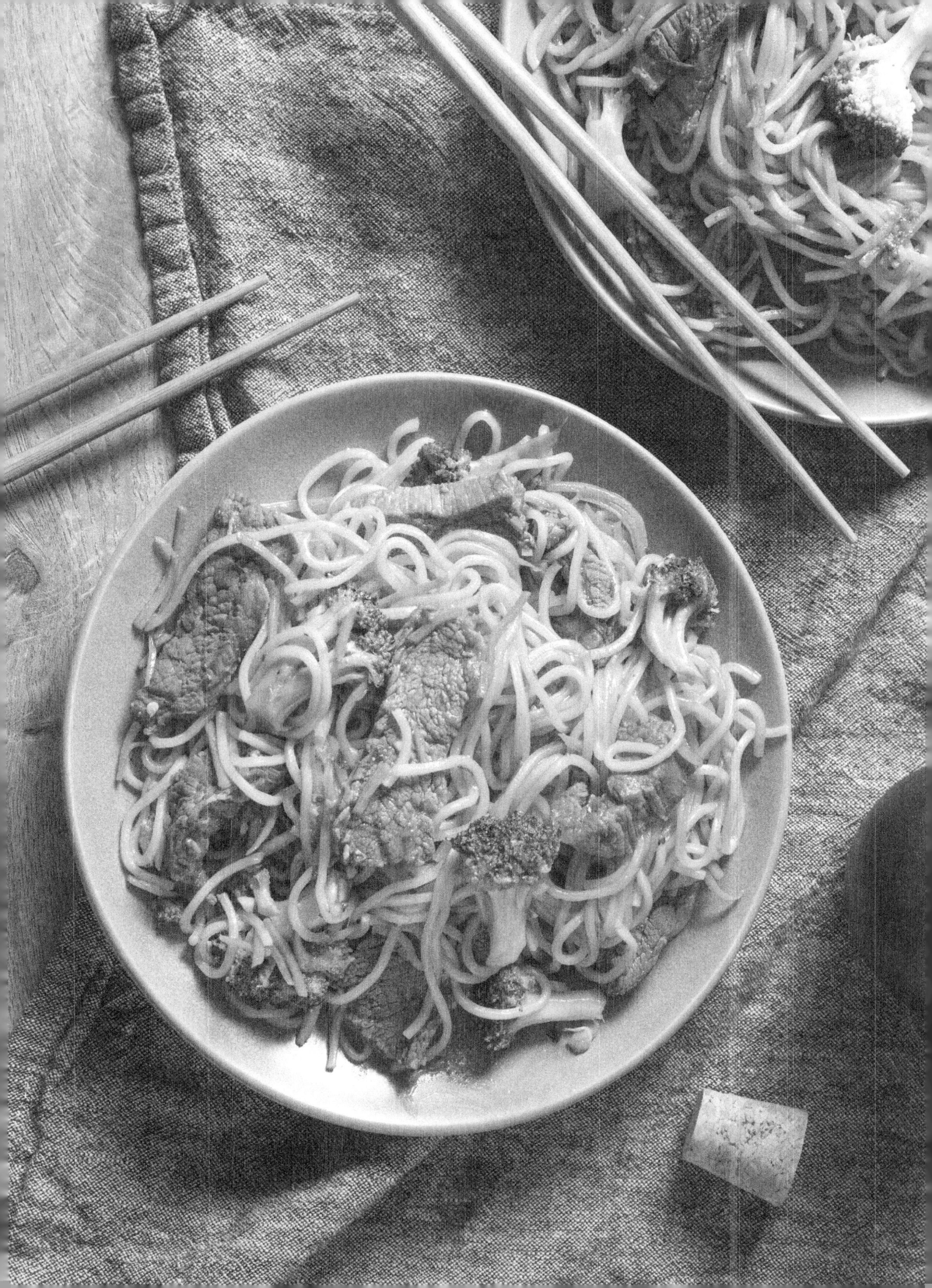

HOISIN BEEF NOODLE

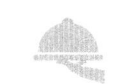

SERVINGS - 4

TIME - 20 min

 NUTRITIONAL VALUE

- Calories-476kcal
- Carbohydrates-40g
- Proteins-41g
- Fats-18g

 INGREDIENTS

- 1 cup freshly prepared noodles
- 1 tsp sesame oil
- 2 cups lean beef steak
- 2 tbsp Hoisin dressing
- 2 sliced spring onions
- 1 chopped green chili
- ½ cup vegetable salad

 INSTRUCTIONS

1. Grease your grilling pan by adding some oil and cook beef steaks on both sides equally. Cut beef pieces into slices and set them aside.
2. Boil freshly prepared noodles into the water and drain them.
3. Prepare your serving bowl by adding noodles and vegetable salad to the bottom. Add beef slices on top along with Hoisin sauce.
4. Drizzle over some sesame oil along with some spring onions and green chili.

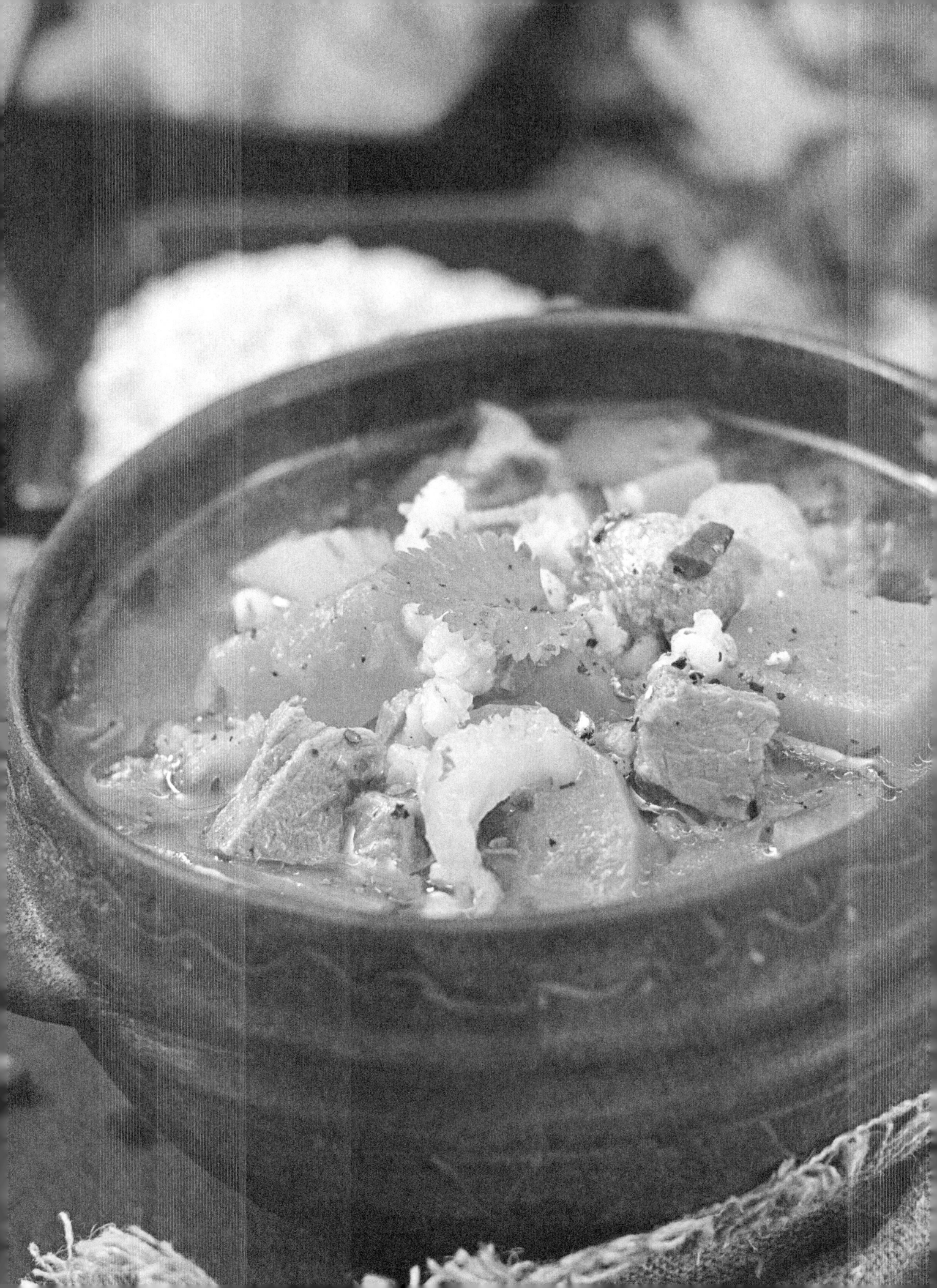

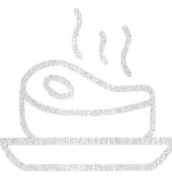

CABBAGE SOUP WITH BEEF

SERVINGS - 8

TIME - 35 min

 NUTRITIONAL VALUE

- Calories-177 kcal
- Carbohydrates-4g
- Proteins-12g
- Fats-15g

 INGREDIENTS

- 2 tbsp olive oil
- 1 chopped onion
- 2 cups rib eye steak
- 1 chopped green cabbage
- 4 minced garlic cloves
- 6 cups beef stock
- 3 tbsp chopped parsley
- 2 tsp dried thyme
- 2 tsp dried rosemary
- 2 tsp onion and garlic powder
- 1 tsp salt
- 1 tsp black pepper

 INSTRUCTIONS

1. Heat oil in a pan and fry beef pieces on medium flame. Also, add some chopped onions into it.
2. Add celery and carrots to the pan. Then add cabbage along with garlic and combine all the ingredients well.
3. Add stock to the pan and add parsley, dried thyme, rosemary, onion, and garlic powder along with some salt.
4. Simmer the contents for 20 minutes and serve with an extra garnish of dried herbs.

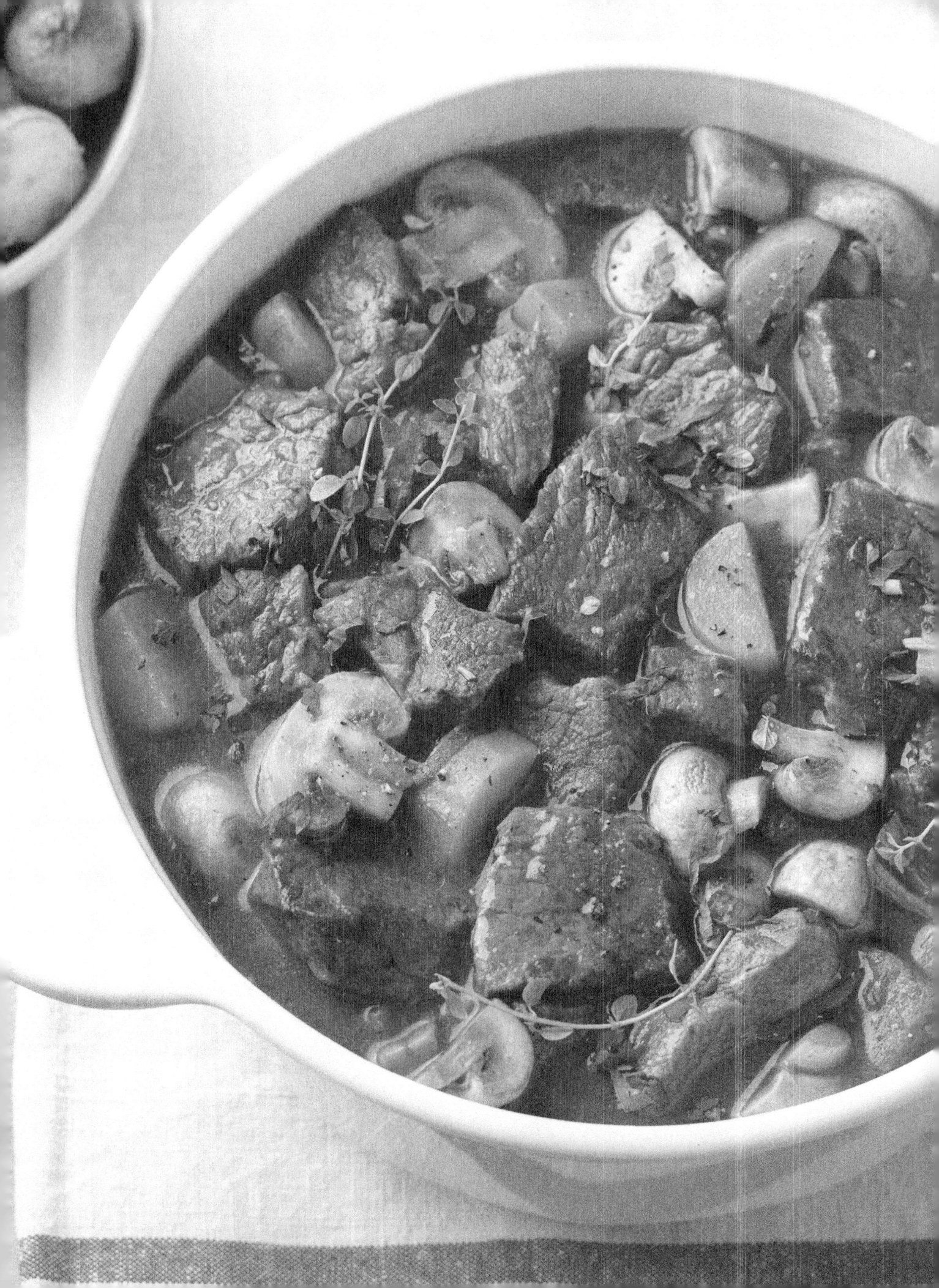

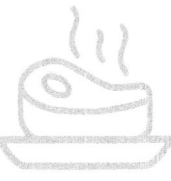

BEEF BOURGUIGNON

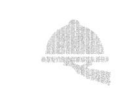

SERVINGS - 6

TIME - 3 Hrs

 NUTRITIONAL VALUE

- Calories-673 kcal
- Carbohydrates-17g
- Proteins-56g
- Fats-44g

 INGREDIENTS

- 1 tbsp olive oil
- ½ cup chopped bacon
- 5 cup beef brisket
- 1 sliced carrot
- 1 diced onion
- 6 minced garlic cloves
- 1 tsp salt
- 1 tsp pepper
- 2 tbsp flour
- 3 cups beef stock
- 2 tbsp tomato paste
- 1 tsp thyme
- 2 bay leaves
- ½ cup mushrooms
- 2 tbsp butter

 INSTRUCTIONS

1. Preheat your oven to 347 degree Fahrenheit (175 degree Celsius).
2. Fry bacon into the oil until crispy and transfer it to a bowl.
3. Grill beef slices on both sides until fully cooked. Set them aside.
4. Take another pan and sauté onions and carrots into it. Then add garlic. Cook for 5 minutes.
5. Add beef and bacon into the pot and also add some seasonings.
6. Add flour and again cook for 10 minutes.
7. After cooking for 10 minutes add beef stock and tomato paste. Bring the pot to simmer the contents.
8. Fry mushrooms separately and add in the beef mixture.
9. Garnish with herbs and serve.

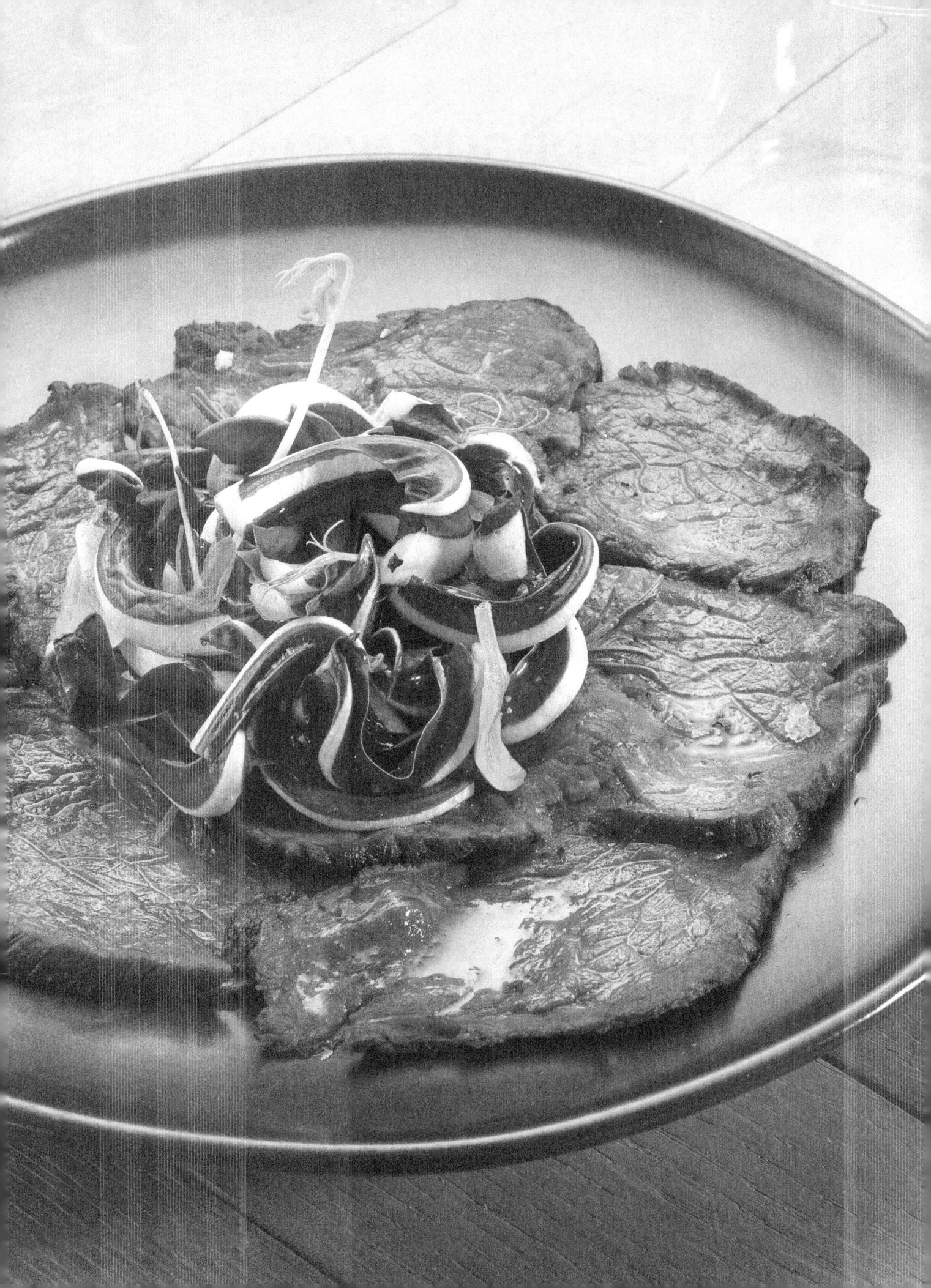

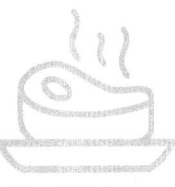

ROASTED BEEF TENDERLOIN

SERVINGS - 8

TIME - 1 hr 10 min

NUTRITIONAL VALUE

- Calories-797 kcal
- Carbohydrates-4g
- Proteins-53g
- Fats-104g

INGREDIENTS

- 8 cups trimmed beef tenderloin pieces
- 3 tsp salt
- 2 tsp black pepper
- 2 tbsp oil
- ½ cup butter
- 4 large minced garlic cloves
- ½ tsp mustard
- 2 tbsp vegetable oil
- 1 chopped onion
- 2 cups beef broth
- 1 tsp thyme

INSTRUCTIONS

1. Preheat your oven to 428 degree Fahrenheit (220 degrees Celsius).
2. Season your tenderloin by adding salt and pepper.
3. Sear both sides of tenderloin by frying the pieces into a pan at medium flame.
4. In a small mixing bowl and butter, garlic and mustard. Apply half of the mixture onto the beef pieces and set aside half.
5. Place pieces of beef glazed with butter onto a baking dish and bake the pieces for 20 minutes.
6. Cut the pieces into smaller ones.
7. To prepare sauce heat vegetable oil in a pan and sauté onions into it. Add thyme and season the onion with pepper and salt.
8. Pour in beef broth and reduce it.
9. Add the remaining half garlic butter mixture into the sauce and serve it with beef tenderloin pieces.

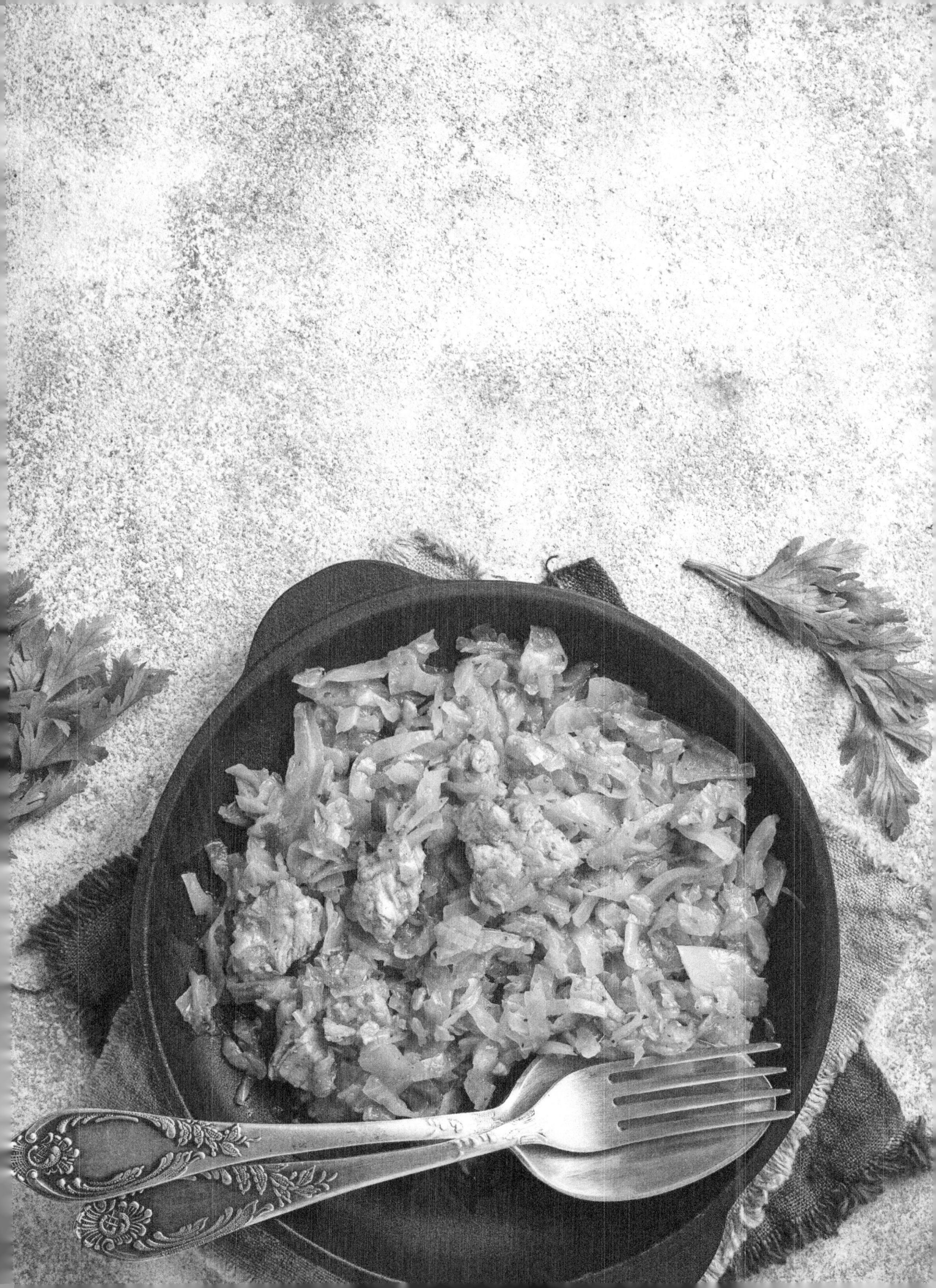

BUTTER BRAISED CABBAGE WITH CRISPY HAM

SERVINGS - 3

TIME - 1 h

 NUTRITIONAL VALUE

- Calories-489 kcal
- Carbohydrates-5g
- Proteins-8.2g
- Fats-48.4g

 INGREDIENTS

- 2 heads of green cabbage
- 1 cup olive oil
- Salt as per taste
- Black pepper as per taste
- 6 slices prosciutto di Parma

 INSTRUCTIONS

1. Take a large pot and add olive oil along with some sliced cabbage into it. Cook it on low heat with constant stirring and put on the lid between the batches of stirring.
2. Place slices of prosciutto di Parma onto a baking dish and season it with some salt and pepper. Bake the slices until they are crispy and crunchy.
3. Crumble the slices and set them aside.
4. To prepare the serving bowl, add cabbage at the bottom and top it with crumbled pieces.

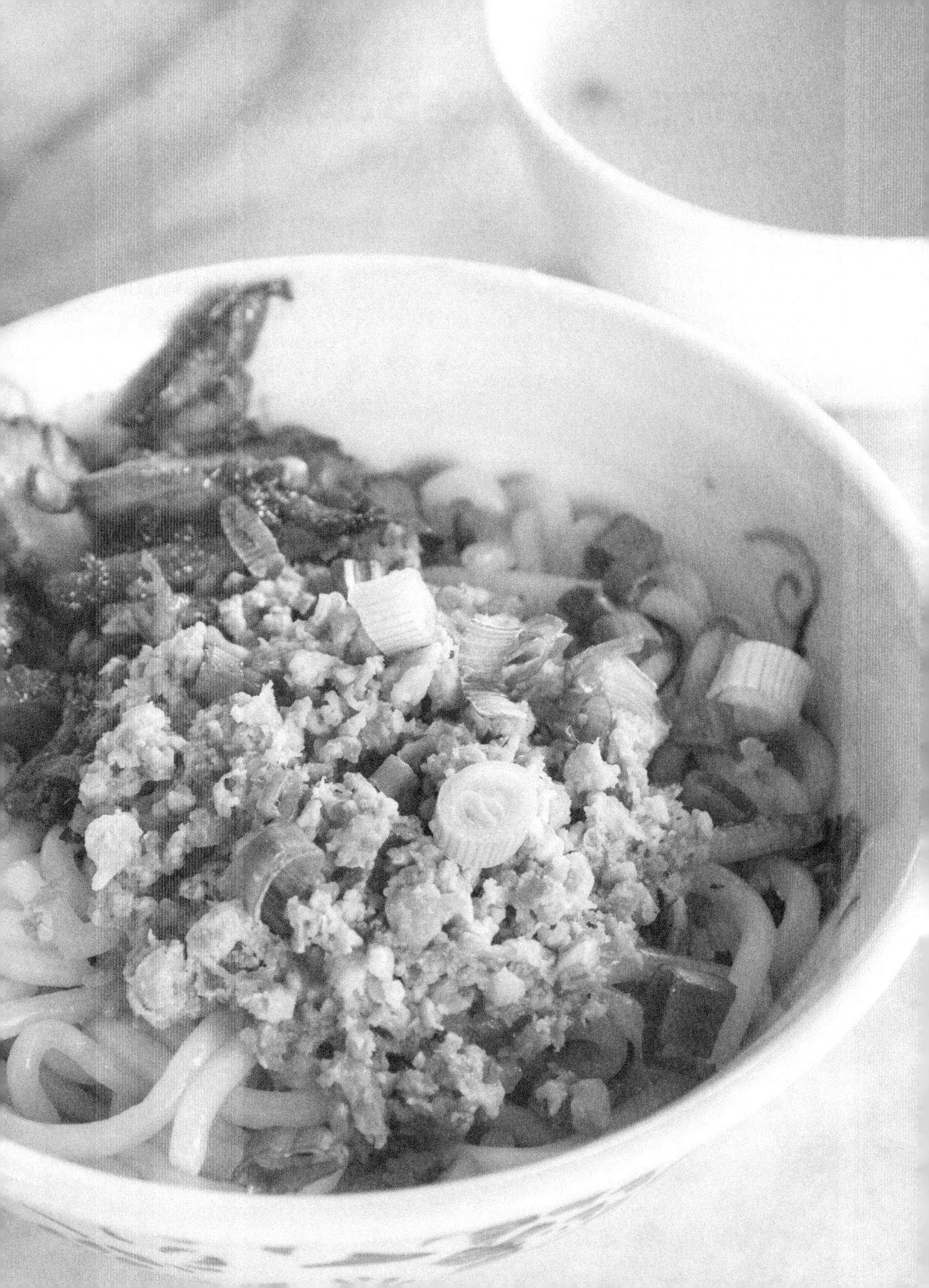

ANUT BUTTER NOODLES WITH CRISPY PORK BELLY

SERVINGS - 2

TIME - 30 min

 NUTRITIONAL VALUE

- Calories- 652 cal
- Carbohydrates-28.7g
- Proteins-59.7g
- Fats-60g

 INGREDIENTS

 INSTRUCTIONS

- 2 cups freshly prepared wheat flour noodles
- 3 tbsp peanut butter
- 1 tbsp rice vinegar
- 2tbsp coconut aminos
- 1 tbsp chili sesame oil
- 3 chopped green onions
- ½ tbsp minced ginger
- ½ tbsp minced garlic
- 1 cup diced pork belly
- 2 tbsp fresh chopped cilantro

1. In a small bowl mix peanut butter, vinegar, water, aminos, and chili sesame oil together. Set it aside.
2. In a pan cook pork belly on medium flame until crispy. Add a few chili sesame oils, coconut aminos, ginger, and garlic. Stir everything together.
3. Boil noodles and add noodles into the pot containing pork. Cook everything for 3 minutes,
4. Scoop out noodle mixture in a bowl and drizzle over peanut butter sauce. Sprinkle some chopped cilantro on top and serve.

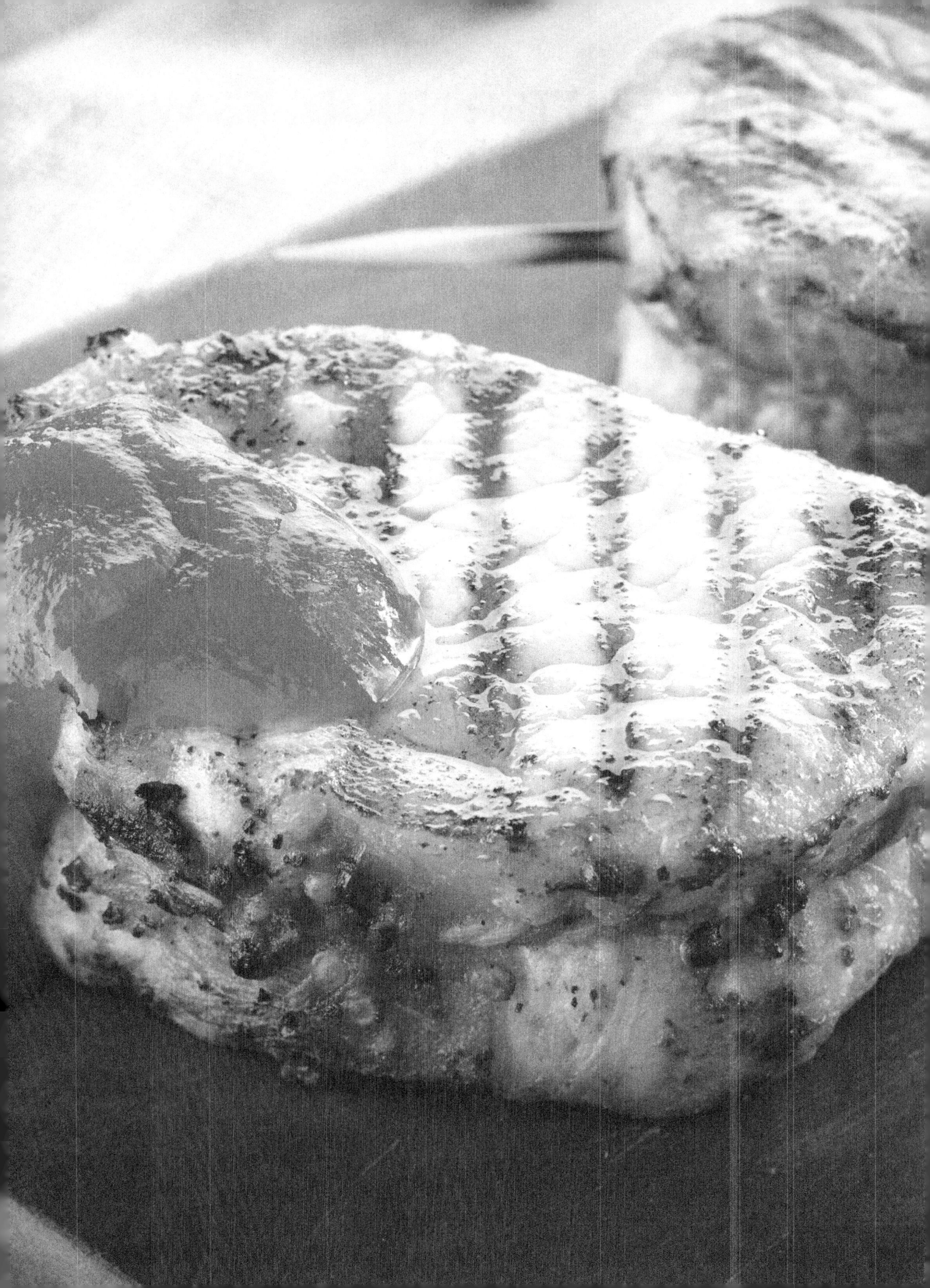

GRILLED PORK TENDERLOIN

SERVINGS - 4

TIME - 30 min

 NUTRITIONAL VALUE

- Calories-141 k cal
- Carbohydrates-0g
- Proteins-23g
- Fats-5g

 INGREDIENTS

- 2 cup pork tenderloin
- 2 tbsp Dijon Mustard
- 1 tsp salt
- 1 tsp black pepper

 INSTRUCTIONS

1. In a small mixing bowl add Dijon mustard, salt, and pepper.
2. Apply the mixture to the pork tenderloin and grill the pieces onto the grill pan and serve with a sauce.

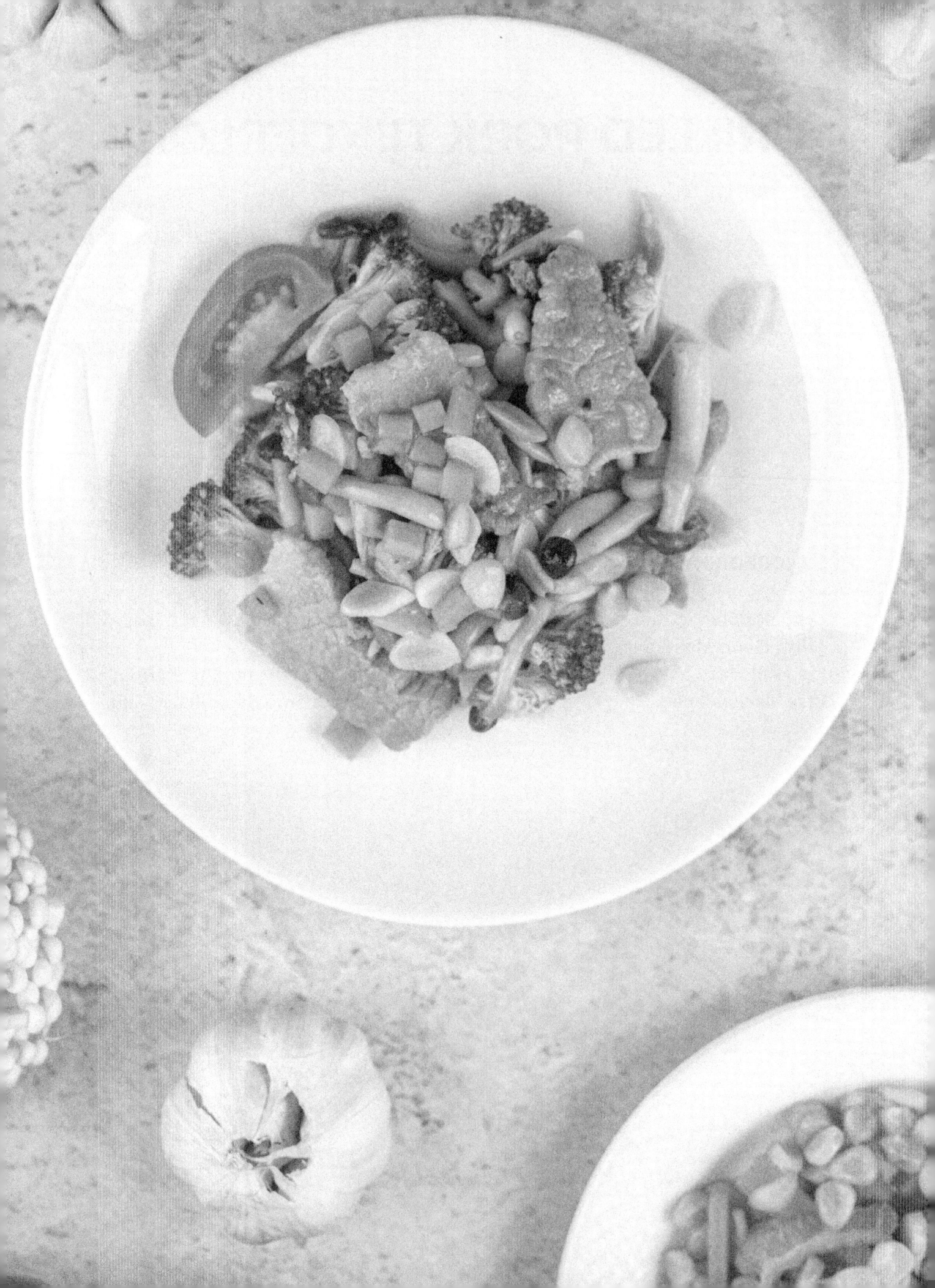

PORK STIR FRY

SERVINGS - 4

TIME - 15 min

 NUTRITIONAL VALUE

- Calories-226kcal
- Carbohydrates-10g
- Proteins-19g
- Fats-12g

 INGREDIENTS

 INSTRUCTIONS

- 3 cup of pork loin strips
- 2 tbsp oil
- 1 tbsp minced ginger
- 1 tsp minced garlic
- 1 cup broccoli florets
- 1 diced red bell pepper
- 1 cup green onions
- 2 tbsp soy sauce
- 1 tbsp brown sugar
- 1 tsp cornstarch
- 1 tsp sesame oil

1. Take a pan and oil in it. Add pork strips and cook them until half done.
2. Add vegetables and cook them for 1 minute.
3. Stir fry both contents and add sauces at the end.
4. Mix everything and serve.

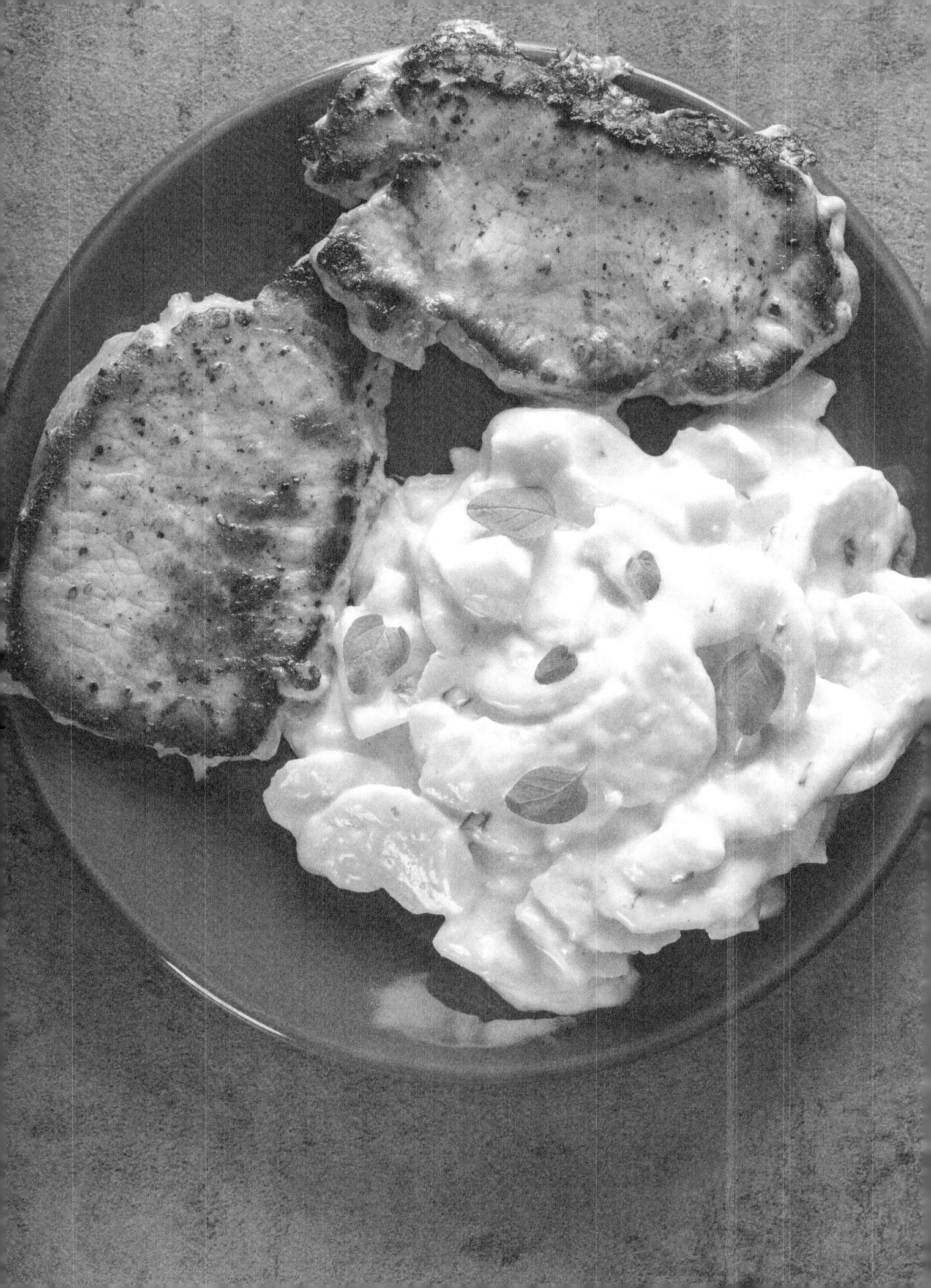

OVEN-FRIED PORK CHOPS

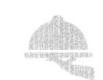

SERVINGS - 4

TIME - 30 min

 NUTRITIONAL VALUE

- Calories-194 kcal
- Carbohydrates-12g
- Proteins-22g
- Fats-8g

 INGREDIENTS

- Cooking spray
- ¼ cup all-purpose flour
- 1 beaten egg
- 1 tsp mustard
- ¾ cup bread crumbs
- 1 tsp ground pepper
- ½ salt
- 1 cup pork chops

 INSTRUCTIONS

1. In a small mixing bowl add mustard and egg together.
2. On another flat plate mix bread crumbs with salt and pepper.
3. Preheat oven to 425 degrees Fahrenheit (200 degrees Celsius).
4. Dip pork chops into the egg mixture and then coat into bread crumbs mixture.
5. Prepare all the chops like this.
6. Add chops into a greased baking dish and cook for 20 minutes.

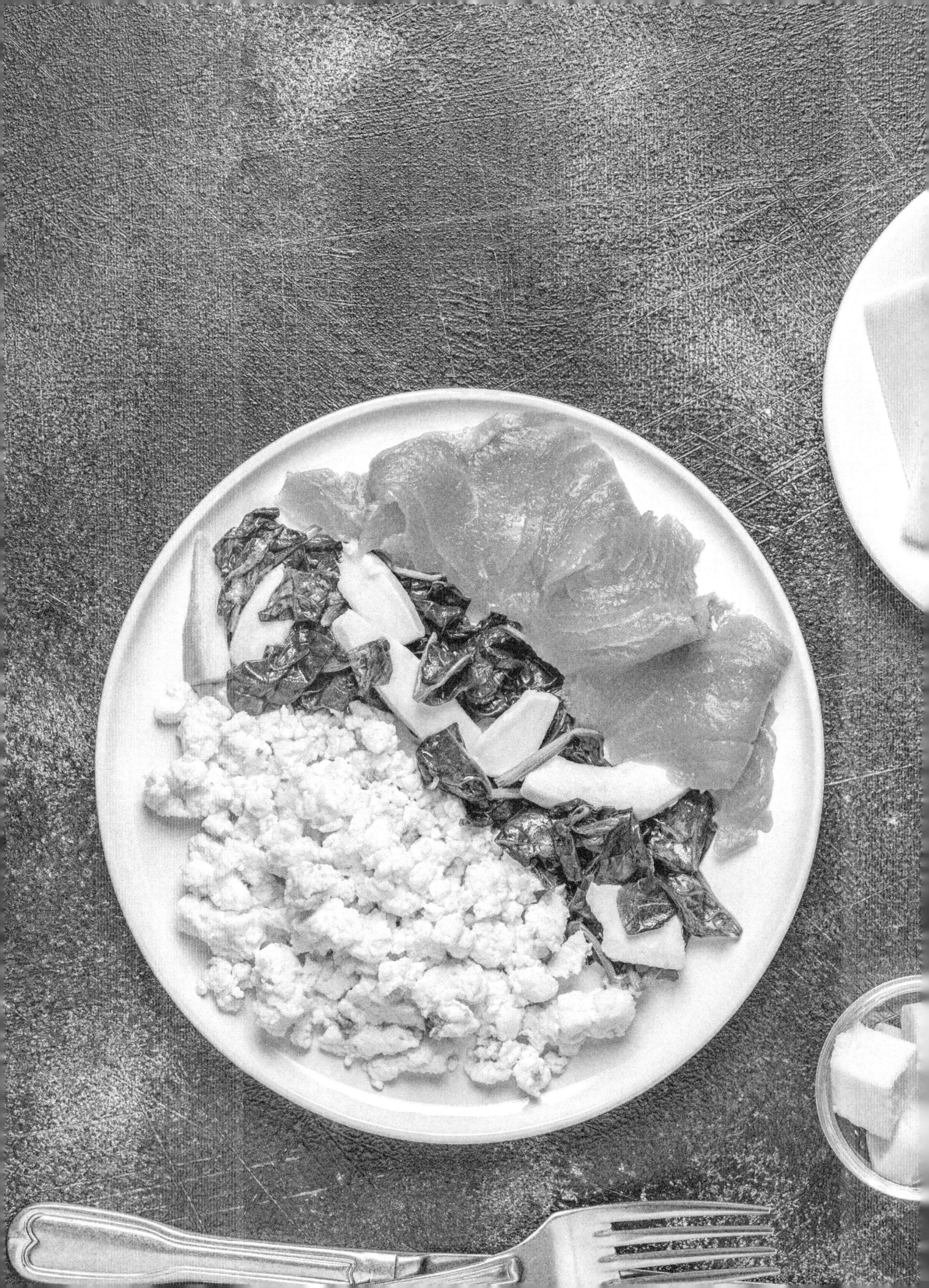

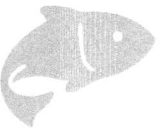

GREEN EGGS WITH SMOKED SALMON

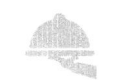

SERVINGS - 1

TIME - 20 min

 NUTRITIONAL VALUE

- Calories- 654 kcal
- Carbohydrates- 2.6 g
- Proteins- 41.4g
- Fats-51.8g

 INGREDIENTS

- 1/3 cup spinach
- 1 tbsp butter
- 3 large eggs
- Salt as per taste
- Black pepper as per taste
- 3 smoked salmon slices
- 1 tbsp chopped chives
- 1 tbsp olive oil

 INSTRUCTIONS

1. Chop the spinach leaves and add them to beaten eggs. Season the egg mixture with some salt and black pepper.
2. Heat the pan and add the egg mixture into it. With the help of a wooden spoon break the egg mixture into crumbled pieces.
3. Prepare your serving plate by placing the scrambled egg and smoked salmon slices onto the plate.
4. Drizzle some chives along with some olive oil and serve.

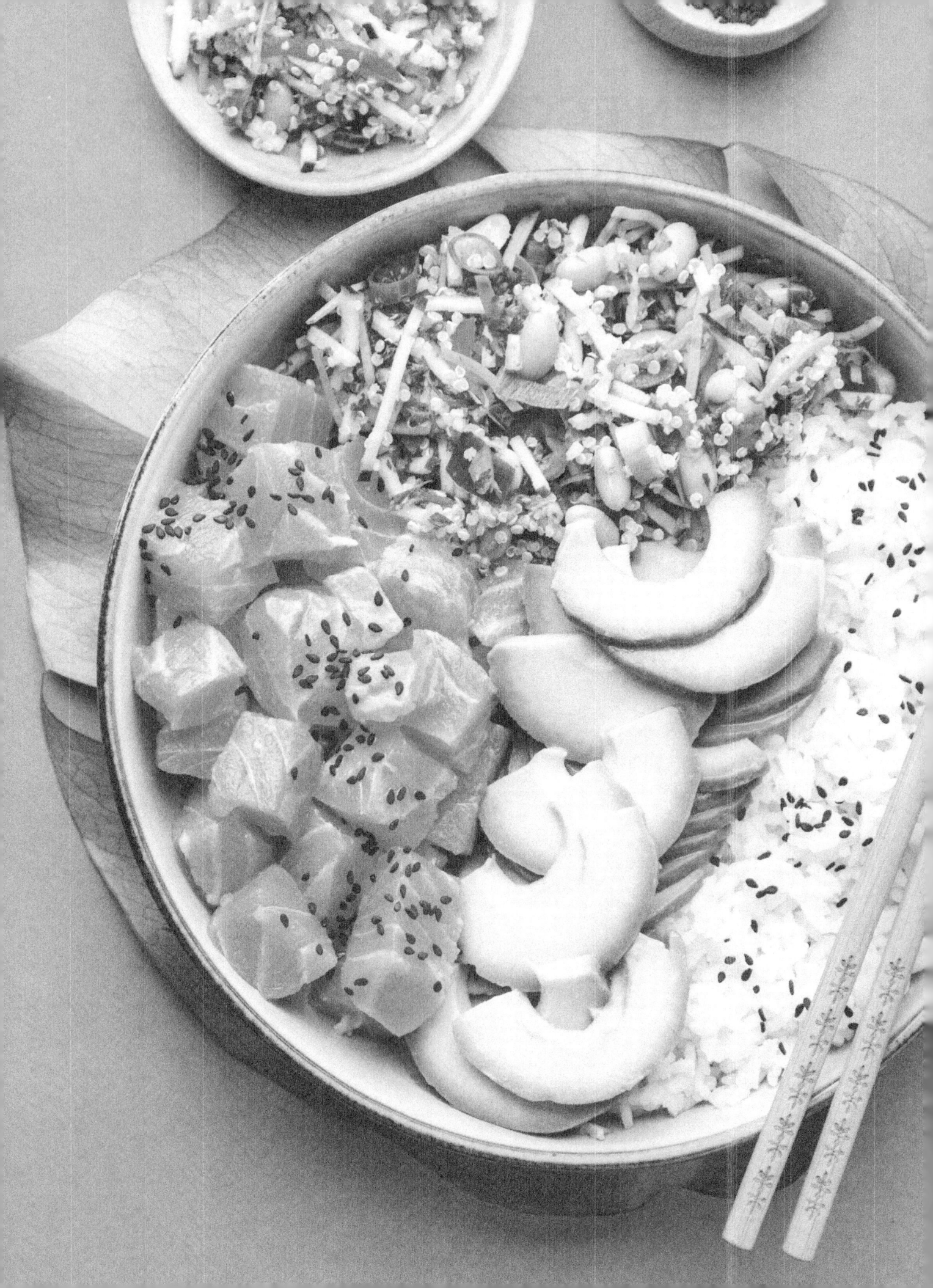

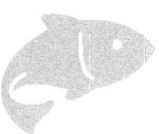

SALMON POWER BOWL

SERVINGS - 2

TIME - 20 min

NUTRITIONAL VALUE

- Calories-537 kcal
- Carbohydrates-4.6 g
- Proteins- 36g
- Fats-39.6g

INGREDIENTS

INSTRUCTIONS

- 1 cup smoked salmon fillet
- ½ sliced avocado
- 2 hard-boiled eggs cut into 4 pieces
- 2tbsp pickled red onion
- 1/3 cup asparagus
- 2 tbsp pumpkin seeds
- 1cup of lettuce

Horseradish Mayonnaise

- 2 tbsp paleo mayonnaise
- 1 tbsp olive oil
- 1 tbsp vinegar
- 1 tbsp horseradish
- ½ tbsp chopped capers
- 1 tbsp parsley
- Salt as per taste
- Black pepper as per taste

1. Prepare Horseradish by combing all the ingredients in a mixing bowl.
2. To prepare the salad bowl, first, boil the asparagus sticks in a water boiler for 7 minutes until they are crispy and crunchy.
3. Add all the remaining ingredients to a serving plate including smoked salmon fillets and fresh greens.
4. Drizzle some mayonnaise over the power bowl and serve.

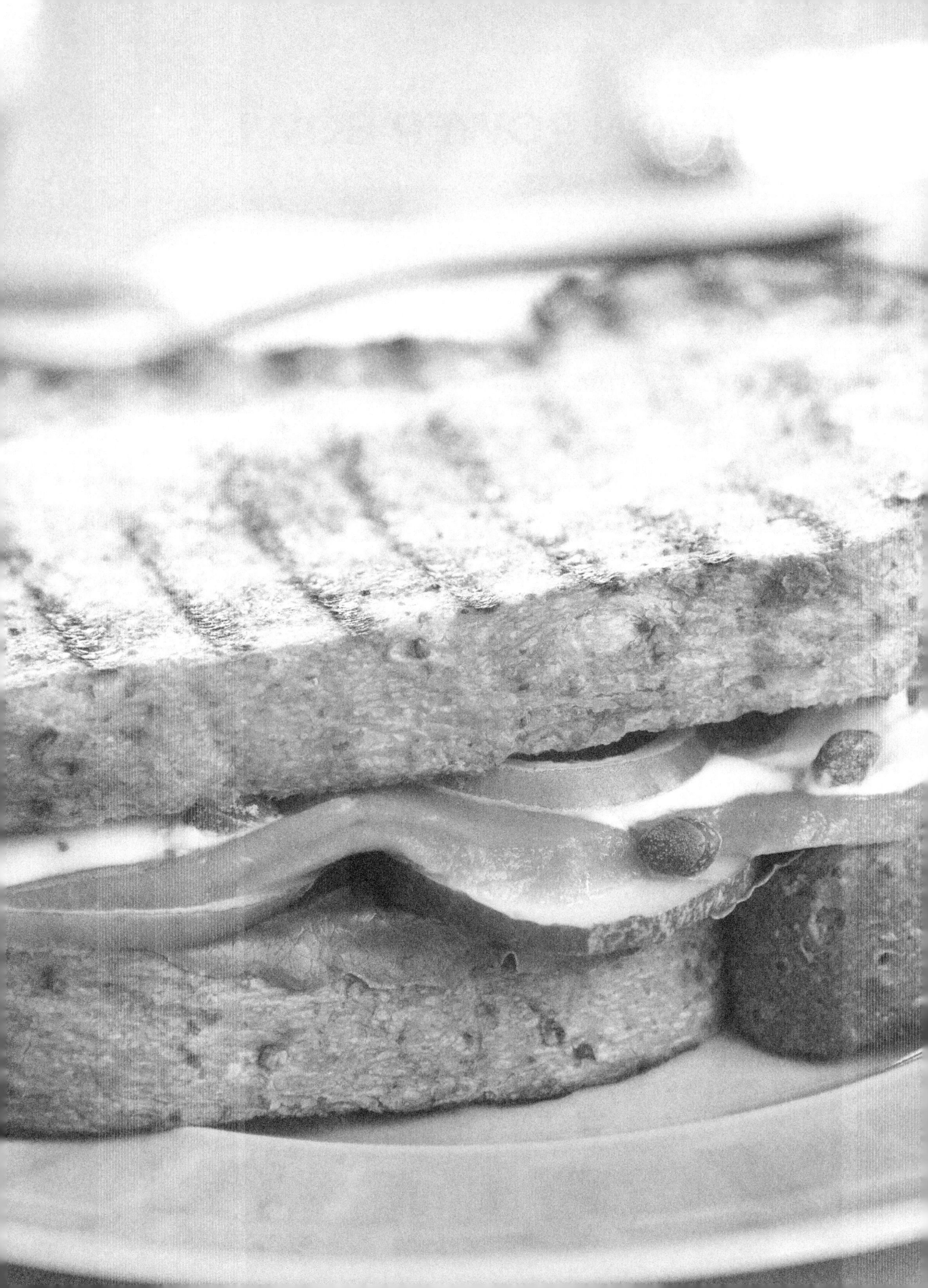

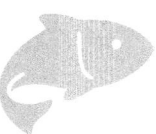

SALMON SANDWICH

SERVINGS - 1

TIME - 30 min

 NUTRITIONAL VALUE

- Calories-789 kcal
- Carbohydrates-5.8g
- Proteins-43.8g
- Fats-64.3g

 INGREDIENTS

- 1 freshly prepared wheat flour bun
- ¾ cup salmon fillet
- 1 tbsp avocado oil
- 2 slices bacon
- 2 lettuce leaves
- 1 sliced tomato
- 1 sliced red onion
- 1 tbsp mayonnaise

 INSTRUCTIONS

1. Season the salmon fillet and grill it on the pan. Also crispy up your bacon slices.
2. For assembling, toast the bun slices onto the same pan and apply mayonnaise to both sides. Stuff in some salmon fillets, tomatoes, onions, bacon, and lettuce leaves.
3. Serve it with some salad or dip.

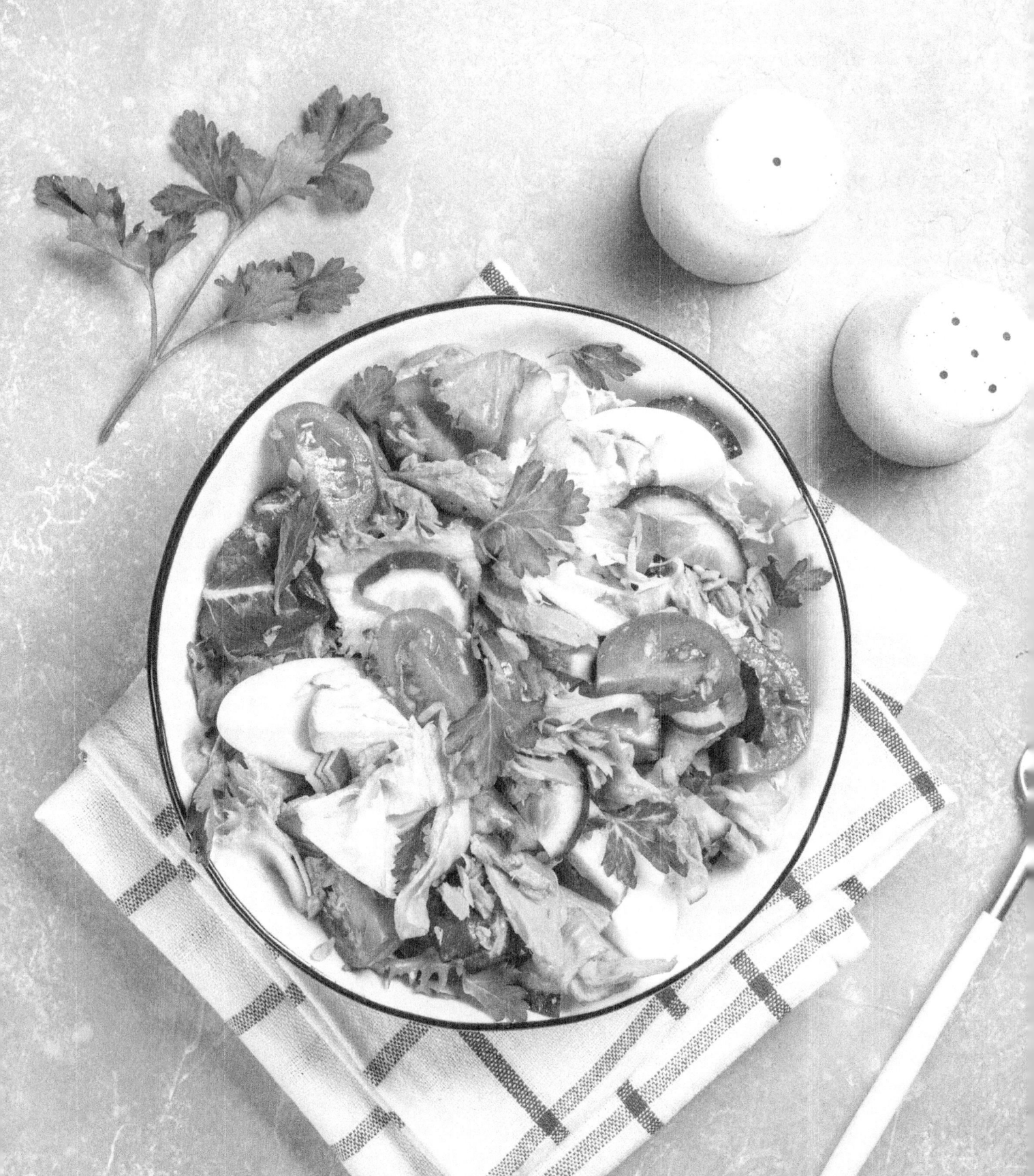

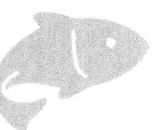

CREAMY PESTO TUNA SALAD

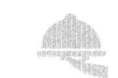

SERVINGS - 1

TIME - 10 min

NUTRITIONAL VALUE

- Calories-698 kcal
- Carbohydrates-7.8g
- Proteins-31.3g
- Fats-58.9g

INGREDIENTS

INSTRUCTIONS

Creamy Tuna
- ½ cup cooked tuna
- 1 ½ tbsp paleo mayonnaise
- 1 tbsp Greek yogurt
- 1 tbsp pesto
- 2 tbsp fresh lemon juice
- Salt as per taste

Dressing
- 1 tbsp olive oil
- ½ tbsp vinegar
- 1/8 tsp salt
- 1/8 tsp black pepper

Salad:
- 4 iceberg lettuce
- 1 sliced tomato
- ½ sliced cucumber
- ¼ sliced avocado

1. Prepare creamy tuna by mixing all the ingredients required for its preparation. Mash tuna pieces with the help of a fork.
2. To prepare dressing take a small jar and mix all the required ingredients into it for dressing.
3. Take an empty bowl and place the veggies at the bottom. Top up with dressing and creamy tuna. Serve fresh.

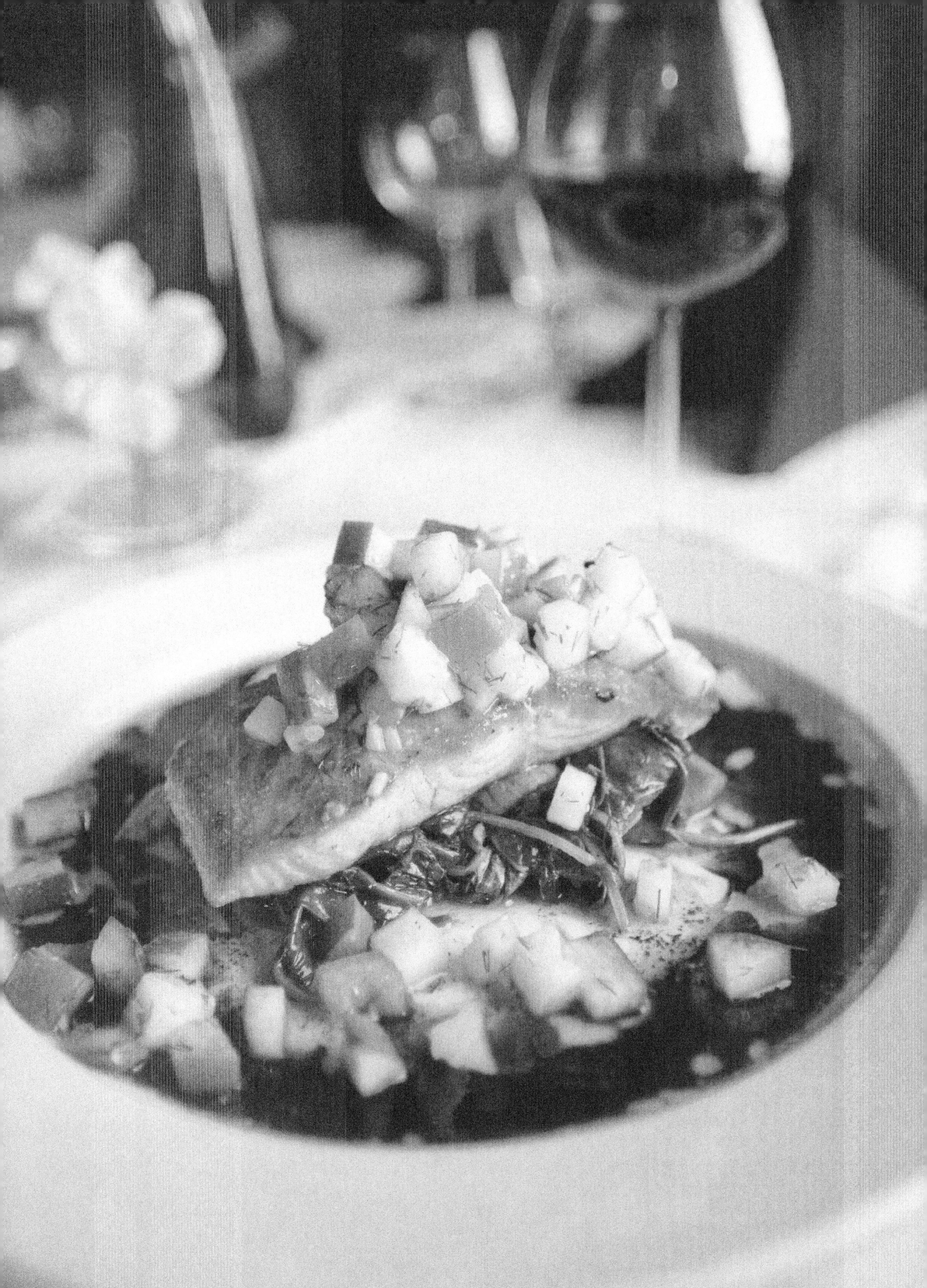

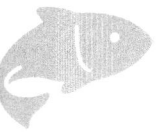

SALMON AND TABBOULEH LOW CARB BOWL

SERVINGS - 2

TIME - 20 min

 NUTRITIONAL VALUE

- Calories-629 kcal
- Carbohydrates-9.6g
- Proteins-42.8g
- Fats-45.2g

 INGREDIENTS

- 2 salmon fillets
- Salt as per taste
- Black pepper as per taste
- 1 tbsp olive oil
- ½ cauliflower
- ½ cup shredded cabbage
- ¼ cup chopped sugar snap peas
- 1/3 cup chopped red pepper
- ¼ cup sliced onion
- ¼ cup chopped parsley
- 2 tbsp chopped mint
- ½ cup crumbled feta
- 3 tbsp olive oil
- 2 tsp fresh lemon juice

Basil Yogurt Dressing
- 1 tbsp Greek yogurt
- 1 tbsp chopped basil
- 1 tsp lemon juice
- Salt as per taste
- Black pepper as per taste

 INSTRUCTIONS

1. Fry salmon by seasoning it with salt, pepper, and olive oil. fry it onto a pan or in the oven.
2. Crush the cauliflower florets in a food processor until they acquire the shape of rice.
3. In another bowl mix, olive oil, lemon juice, salt, and pepper. It's your dressing.
4. To the cauliflower rice add the chopped cabbage, sugar snap peas, and onion, red pepper, and fresh herbs.
5. Add the dressing along with some crumbled feta cheese to the cauliflower rice bowl.
6. To prepare basil yogurt dressing mix all the required ingredients.
7. Add basil yogurt dressing to the cauliflower rice bowl and put a piece of salmon on top.

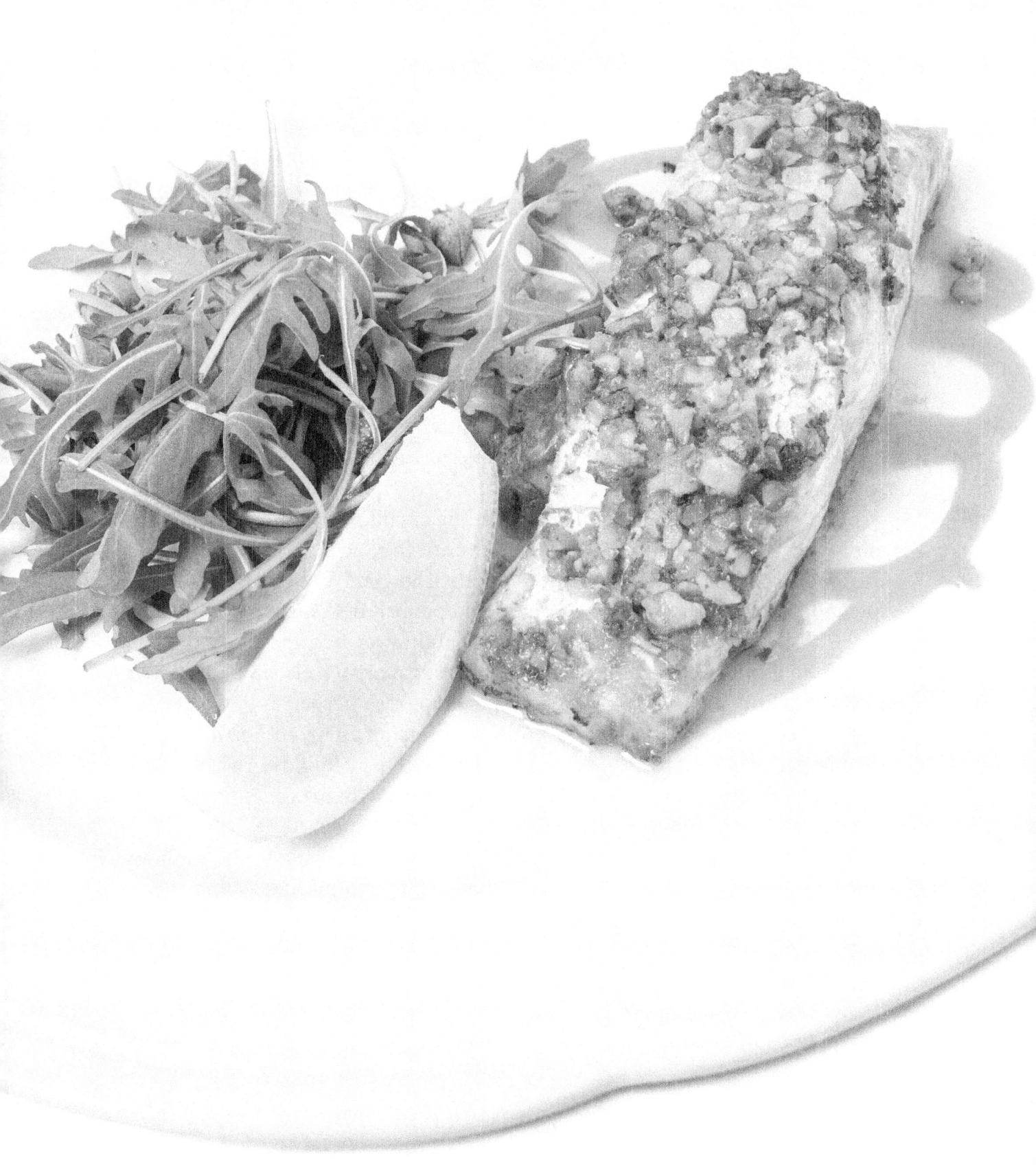

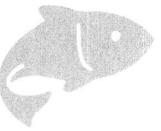

WALNUT ROSEMARY CRUSTED SALMON

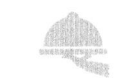

SERVINGS - 2

TIME - 25 min

 NUTRITIONAL VALUE

- Calories- 222 kcal
- Carbohydrates-10.8g
- Proteins-53.7g
- Fats- 26.3g

 INGREDIENTS

- 2 tsp mustard
- 1 minced garlic clove
- ¼ tsp lemon zest
- 1 tsp lemon juice
- 1 tsp rosemary
- ½ tsp kosher salt
- ¼ tsp red chili powder
- 3 tbsp bread crumbs
- 3 tbsp chopped walnuts
- 1 tsp olive oil
- ½ kg salmon fillet
- Lemon wedges for garnishing

 INSTRUCTIONS

1. In a large bowl add mustard, garlic clove, lemon zest, lemon juice, rosemary, salt, red chili, bread crumbs, and walnuts. Combine all the ingredients and set them aside.
2. Now take salmon fillets and coat them in the above mixture.
3. Preheat your oven at at 473 degrees Fahrenheit (245 degrees Celsius) and line up a baking sheet.
4. Grease your baking sheet with the help of a cooking spray and place salmon fillets on top of each sheet.
5. Bake fillets for 10 minutes and garnish them with lemon wedges.

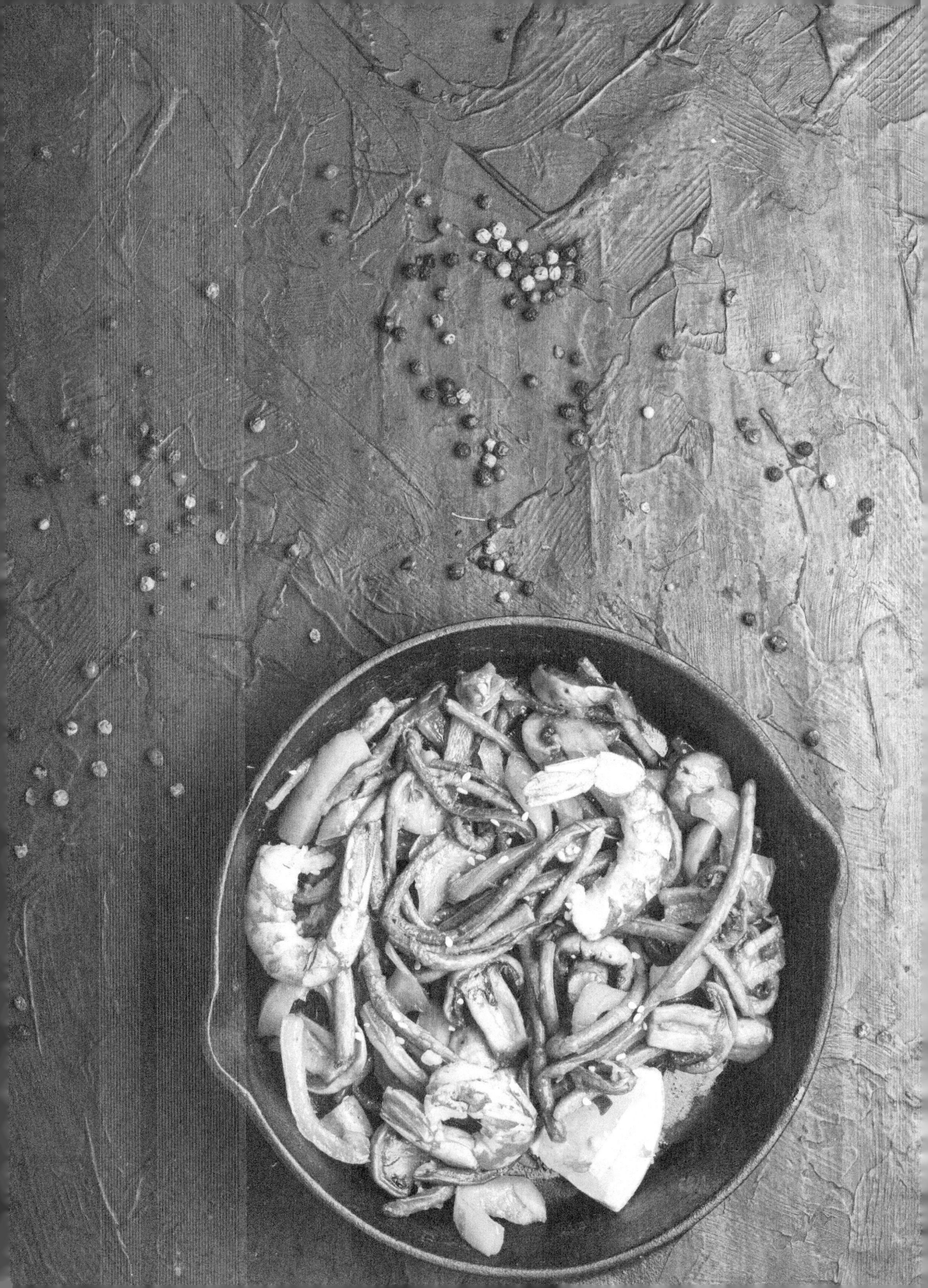

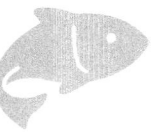

PRAWNS WITH PINEAPPLE AND GREEN BEANS

SERVINGS - 2

TIME - 20 min

 NUTRITIONAL VALUE

- Calories-228 kcal
- Carbohydrates-20g
- Proteins-22g
- Fats-7g

 INGREDIENTS

- 1 tbsp vegetable oil
- 2 chopped lemongrass stalks
- 1 tbsp shredded ginger
- ½ cup pineapple chunks
- ½ cup cherry tomatoes
- 1 cup prawns
- 2 basil leaves
- 4 tbsp lime juice
- 2 tbsp chicken stock
- 1 tbsp fish sauce
- 1 tbsp honey

 INSTRUCTIONS

1. In a pan add lemongrass and ginger and sauté them until golden brown.
2. To the same pan add pineappe chunks, beans, cherry tomatoes and fry them for 5 minutes.
3. Add prawns to the above mixture and cook them until they are fully done.
4. Drizzle some basil leaves and serve.

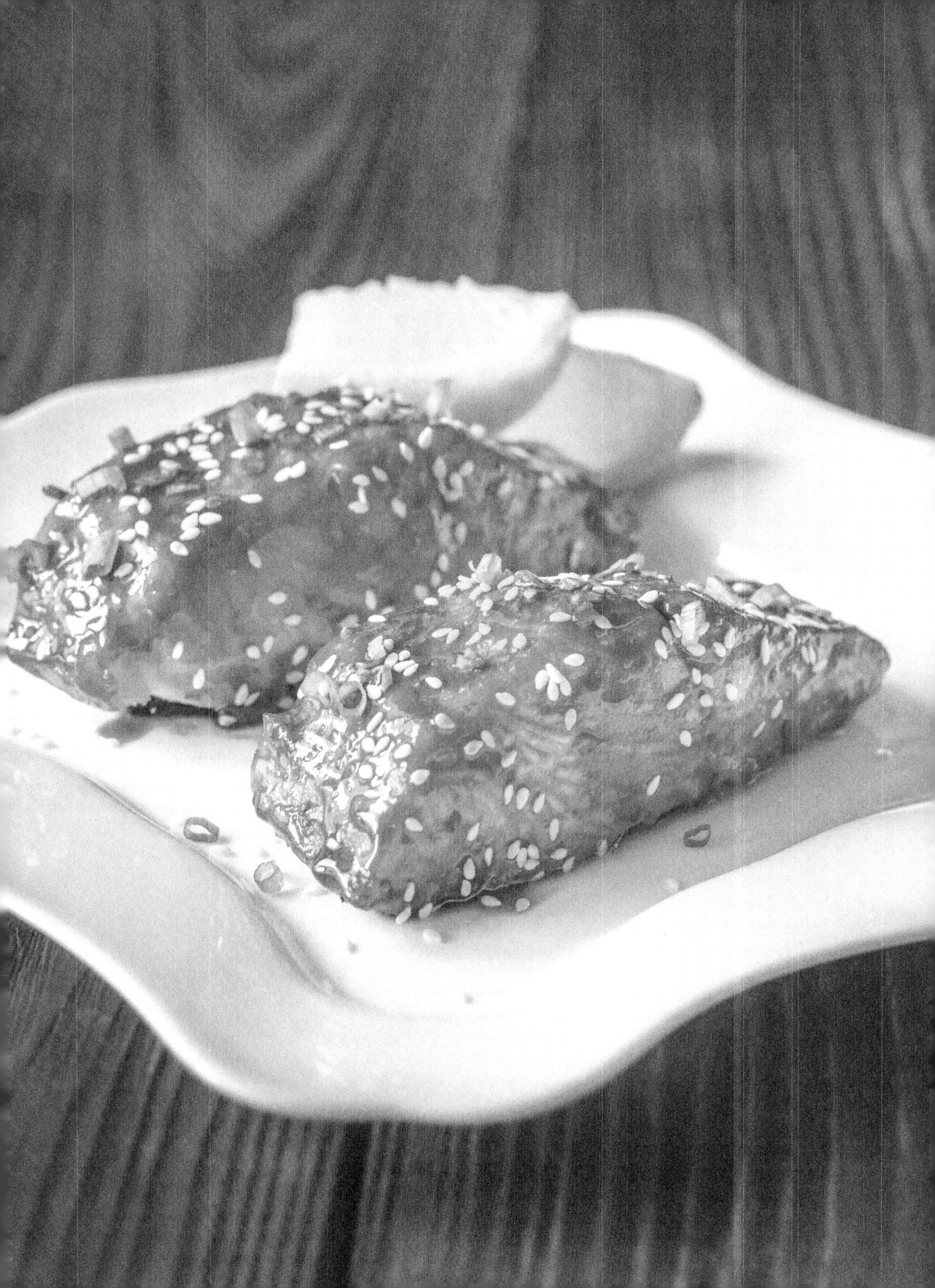

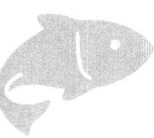

TERIYAKI SALMON PARCELS

SERVINGS - 4

TIME - 20 min

 NUTRITIONAL VALUE

- Calories-243 kcal
- Carbohydrates-8g
- Proteins-24g
- Fats-12g

 INGREDIENTS

- 2 tbsp low-salt soy sauce
- 1 tbsp honey
- 1 minced garlic clove
- 1 cup broccoli
- 2 cups salmon filet
- 1 tsp ginger
- 2 tsp spring onions
- 1 tsp sesame seeds

 INSTRUCTIONS

1. Make 4 squares of 30 cm from aluminum foil. Brush these foil pieces with oil. Raise the edges up a little.
2. Place broccoli stems on foil pieces being topped with a salmon filet and a little drizzle of ginger.
3. Also drizzle some sauce, honey, and sesame seeds. Fold over the edges of the foil and seal them.
4. Put them in a baking dish and place them in an oven heated at 400 degree Fahrenheit (200 degrees Celsius) for 15 minutes.
5. Open the parcels when they need to be served. Garnish with spring onions.

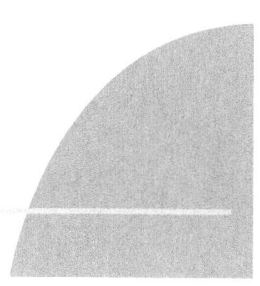

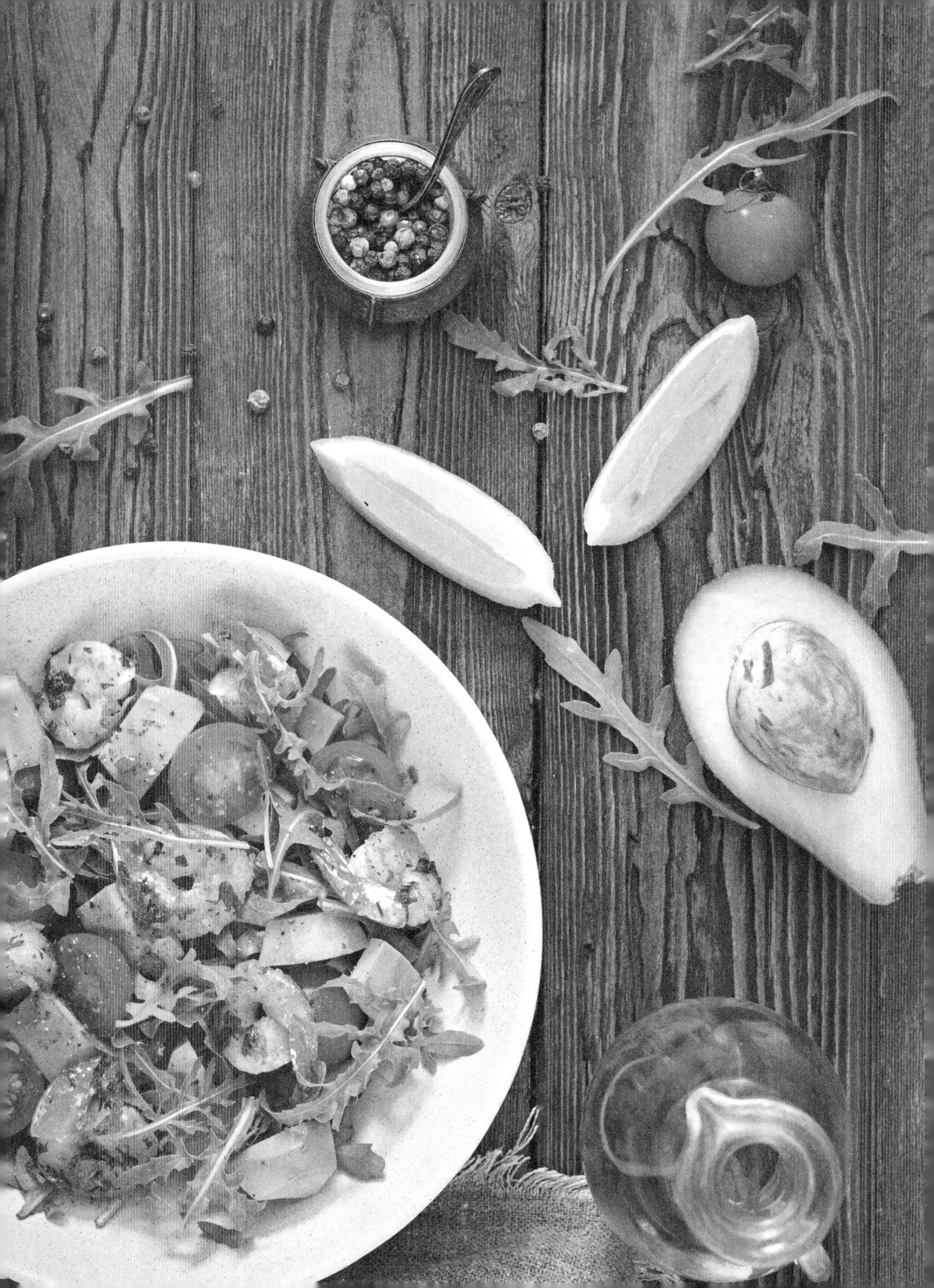

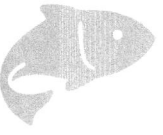

GREEK SHRIMP SOUVLAKI AND FARRO BOWL

SERVINGS - 4

TIME - 45 min

NUTRITIONAL VALUE

- Calories- 467 kcal
- Carbohydrates-54g
- Proteins-34g
- Fats-39g

INGREDIENTS

- ¼ cup olive oil
- 2+1 tbsp lemon juice
- 1tsp granulated garlic + 2 cloves minced garlic
- ¼ + ¾ tsp sea salt
- ½ cup plain Greek yogurt
- 1 tsp paprika
- 1 tsp dried oregano
- ½ tsp black pepper
- ½ kg deveined shrimp
- 2 sliced zucchinis
- 2 sliced bell peppers
- 1 cup dry farro
- 2 cups vegetable broth
- Herbs for garnishing

INSTRUCTIONS

1. To prepare lemon garlic yogurt, combine Greek yogurt with granulated garlic, 1 tbsp lemon juice, and salt in a mixing bowl. Whisk the mixture by the addition of little water.
2. To prepare marination, take a large bowl and add olive oil, 2tbsp lemon juice, minced garlic, paprika, dried oregano salt, and pepper into it.
3. Divide the marination into two equal parts. In one part marinade, deveined shrimps and in other part add diced and sliced vegetables including zucchinis and bell peppers.
4. Take a skillet and cook shrimps into it by greasing the skillet. Cook until shrimps are soft and tender.
5. Now in the same skillet add marinated vegetables and heat them until fully cooked.
6. To prepare farro, boil farro in broth for 30 minutes.
7. Prepare your serving plate by adding a faro at the bottom. Top up your farro with cooked shrimps and vegetables and finally drizzle some lemon garlic yogurt to enhance the taste.

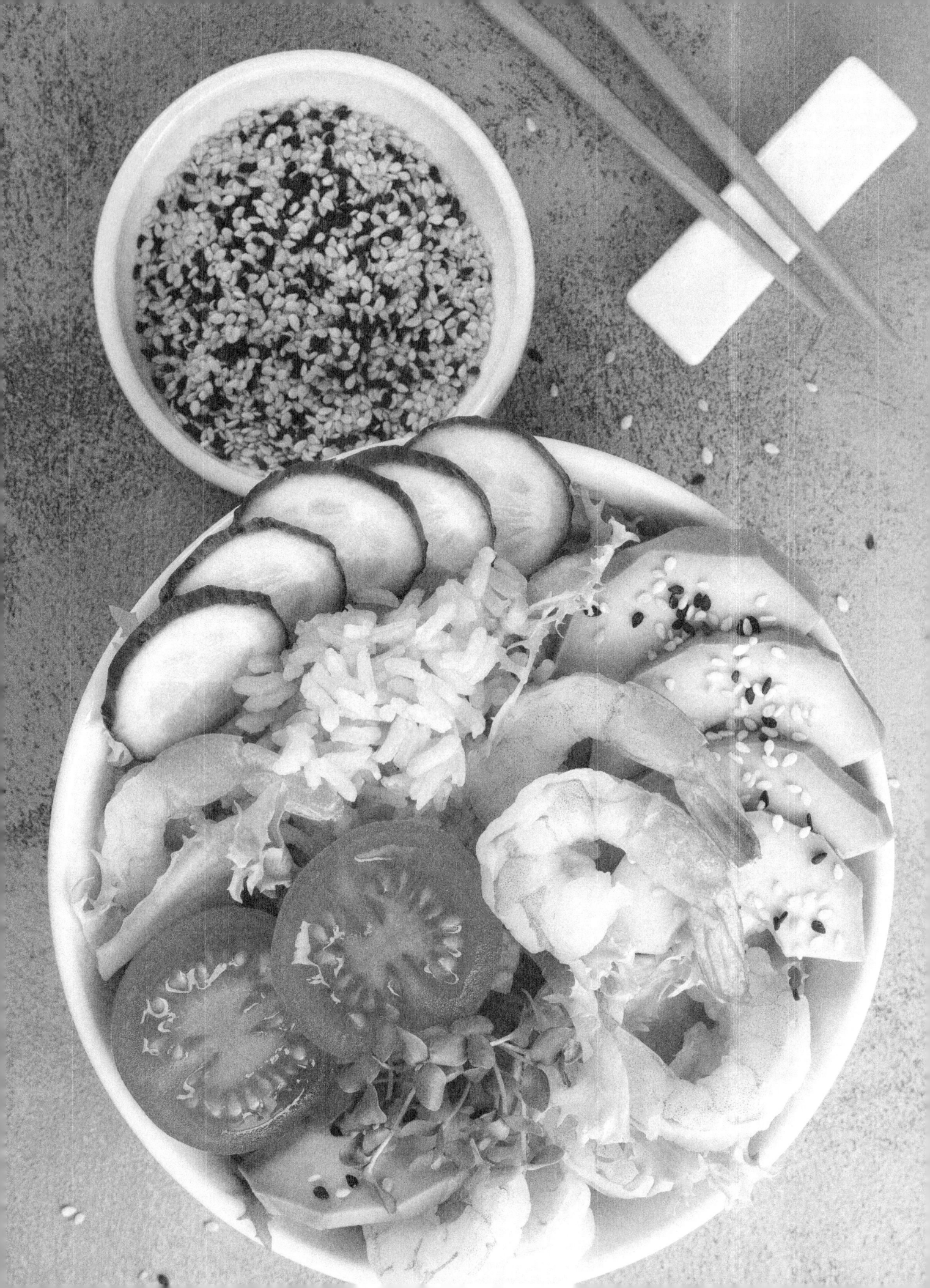

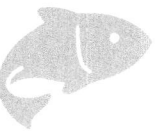

CHARRED SHRIMP PESTO BOWLS

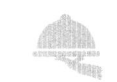

SERVINGS - 2

TIME - 20 min

 NUTRITIONAL VALUE

- Calories-734kcal
- Carbohydrates-83.8g
- Proteins-21.2g
- Fats-39.5g

 INGREDIENTS

- 1/3 cup pesto
- 2 tbsp vinegar
- 1 tbsp olive oil
- 1/3 cup pesto
- 2 tbsp vinegar
- 1 tbsp olive oil
- ½ tsp salt
- ¼ tsp ground black pepper
- ½ kg deveined shrimps
- 4 cups arugula
- 2 cups cooked quinoa
- 1 cup cherry tomatoes
- 1 diced avocado

 INSTRUCTIONS

1. Take a whisking bowl and add pepper, salt, oil, vinegar, and pesto into it. Whisk all the contents of the bowl together to obtain nice consistency.
2. Cook shrimps in a hot pan with a small amount of oil.
3. To prepare serving bowls and arugula with quinoa into it with a bit of vinegar. Top the bowls with tomatoes, avocados, and shrimp.
4. Drizzle the serving bowl with prepared pesto mixture.

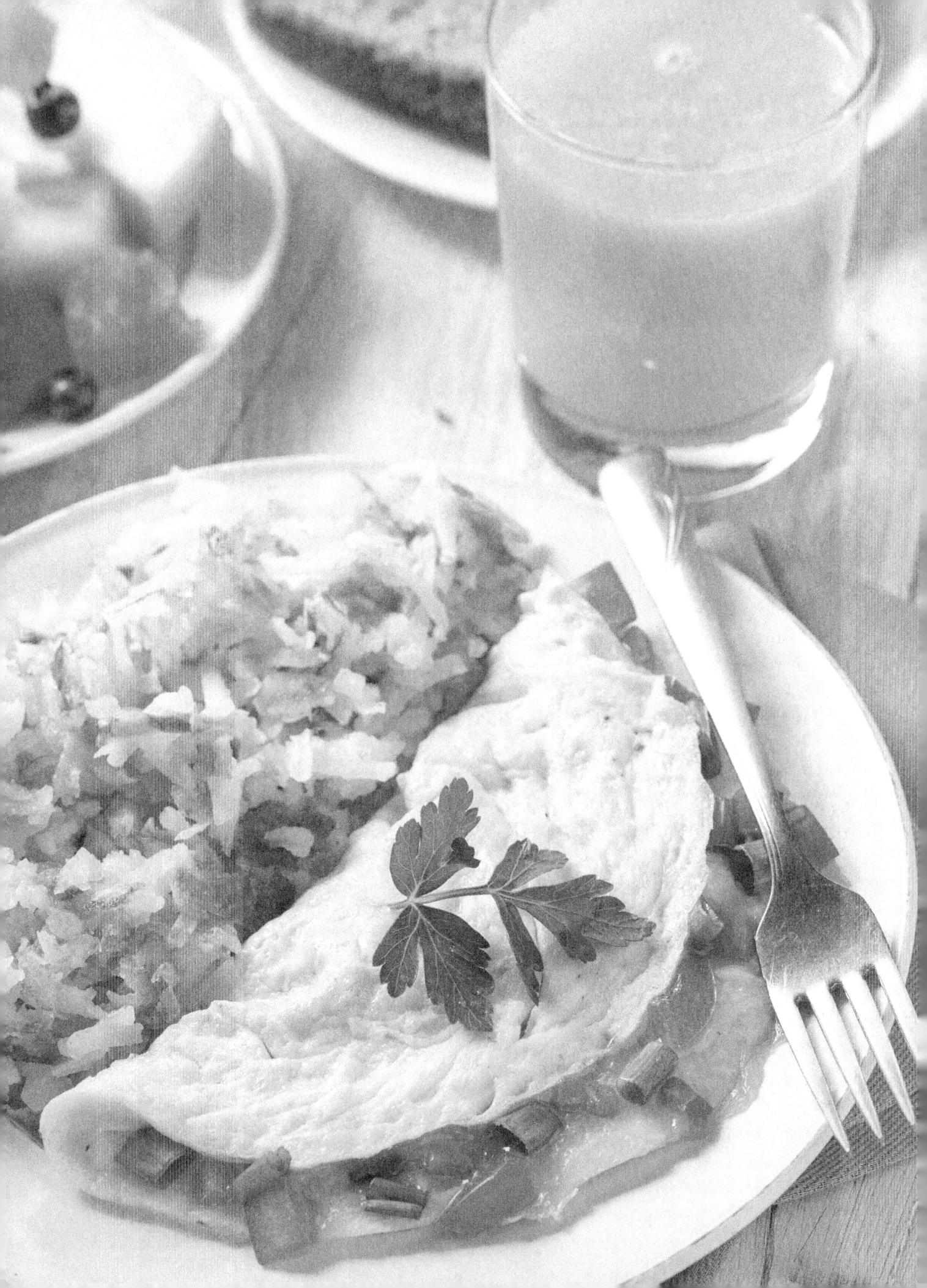

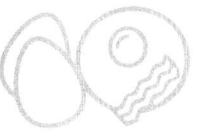

CALIFORNIA OMELET

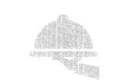

SERVINGS - 3

TIME - 20 min

NUTRITIONAL VALUE

- Calories-615kcal
- Carbohydrates-4.7g
- Proteins-35.4g
- Fats-48.2g

INGREDIENTS

INSTRUCTIONS

- 6 whisked eggs
- ¼ tsp lemon juice
- ¼ tsp Sriracha Sauce
- ¼ tsp salt
- 3 tbsp butter
- 10-12 cooked shrimp pieces
- 2 tbsp chopped cilantro
- ¼ cup minced red bell pepper
- 1 sliced green onion
- 1 sliced avocado
- 2 slices cooked bacon

1. In a large mixing bowl add whisked eggs along with some lemon juice and sriracha sauce.
2. Heat your pan and add a batch of whisked eggs for 1 omelet.
3. Allow the omelet to fry for few minutes.
4. In the omelet add the remaining ingredients and flip the other half of the omelet over to it to close the stuffing.
5. Immediately serve the omelet.

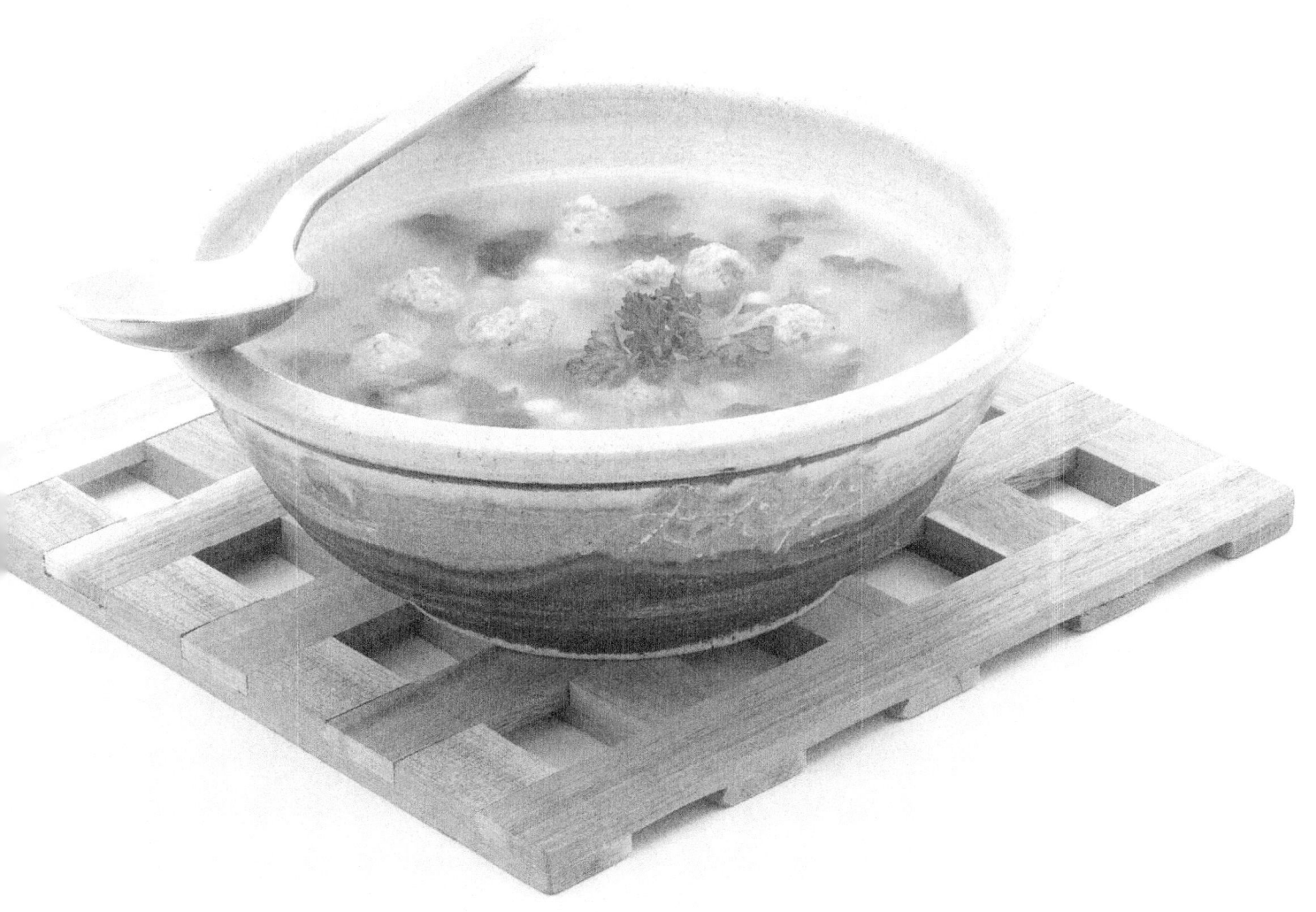

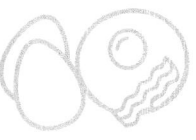

ITALIAN EGG DROP SOUP

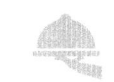

SERVINGS - 3

TIME - 20 min

 NUTRITIONAL VALUE

- Calories-114
- Carbohydrates-1.4g
- Proteins-10.20g
- Fats-7g

 INGREDIENTS

- 4 cups broth
- 4 whole eggs
- ½ cup grated parmesan cheese
- 1 tbsp parsley
- 1 pinch nutmeg
- Salt as per taste
- Pepper as per taste

 INSTRUCTIONS

1. Pour broth into a pot and bring it to a boil.
2. In another bowl add eggs, cheese, nutmeg, parsley, salt, and pepper. Whisk it with the help of a whisker.
3. By continuously stirring the boiling broth add the whisked egg mixture in a thin streamline motion.
4. Cook until little shreds are formed.

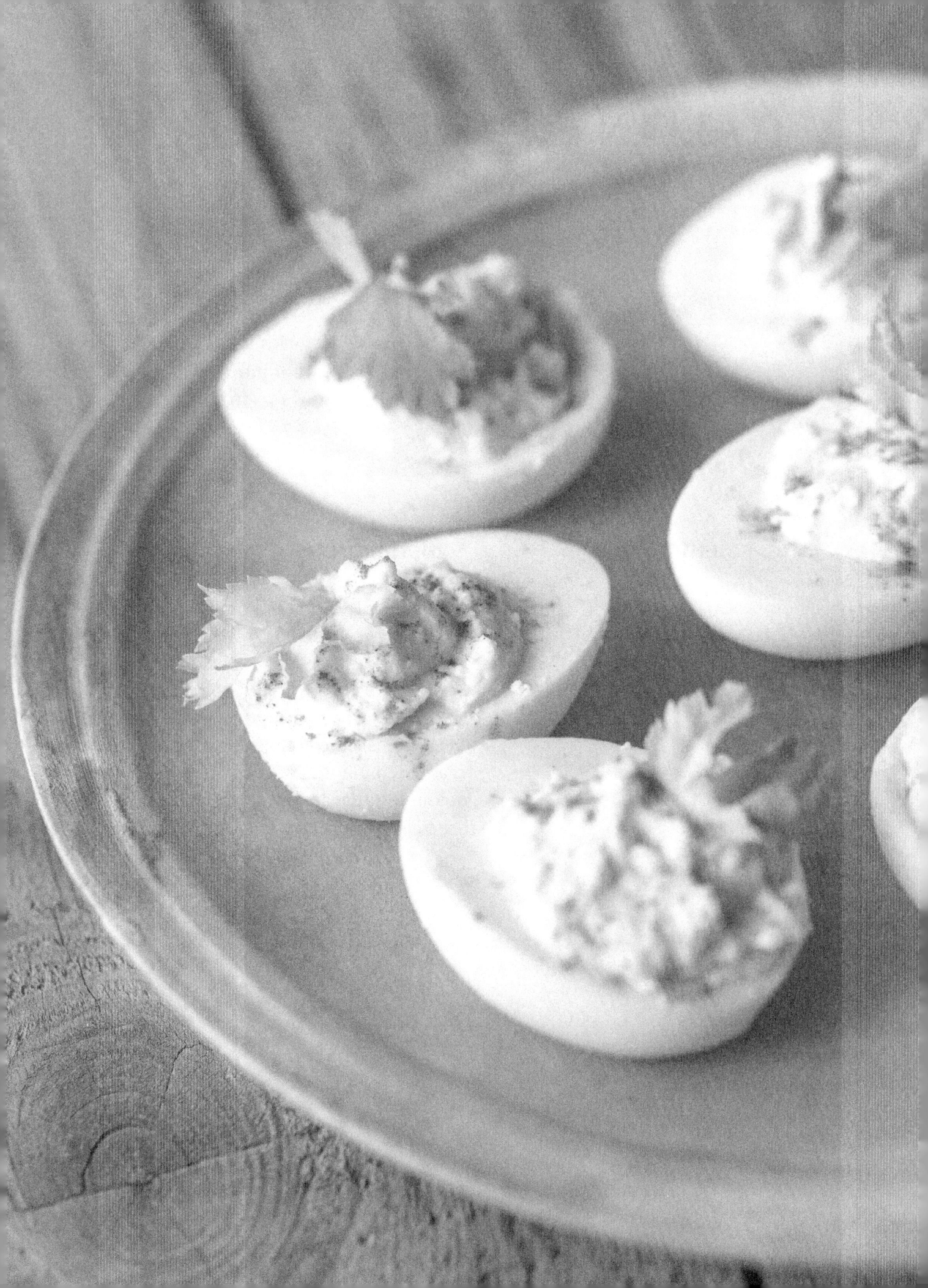

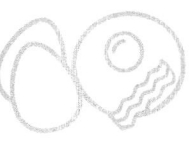

GARLIC DEVIL EGGS

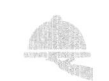

SERVINGS - 6

TIME - 20 min

NUTRITIONAL VALUE

- Calories-137
- Carbohydrates-0.7g
- Proteins-5.6g
- Fats-12.1g

INGREDIENTS

- 6 eggs
- 4 tbsp mayonnaise
- 1 minced garlic clove
- Salt as per taste
- Pepper as per taste
- Chopped parsley

INSTRUCTIONS

1. Boil eggs for 15 minutes until hard-boiled. Peel off the eggshell and cut it into two halves.
2. Separate the yolk from boiled egg whites.
3. Mash egg yolks with mayonnaise, minced garlic, and seasonings. Transfer this mixture into a piping bag with a rosette nozzle on it.
4. Pipe out the egg yolk mixture in the form of small florets onto the egg white cavity and drizzle over some parsley.

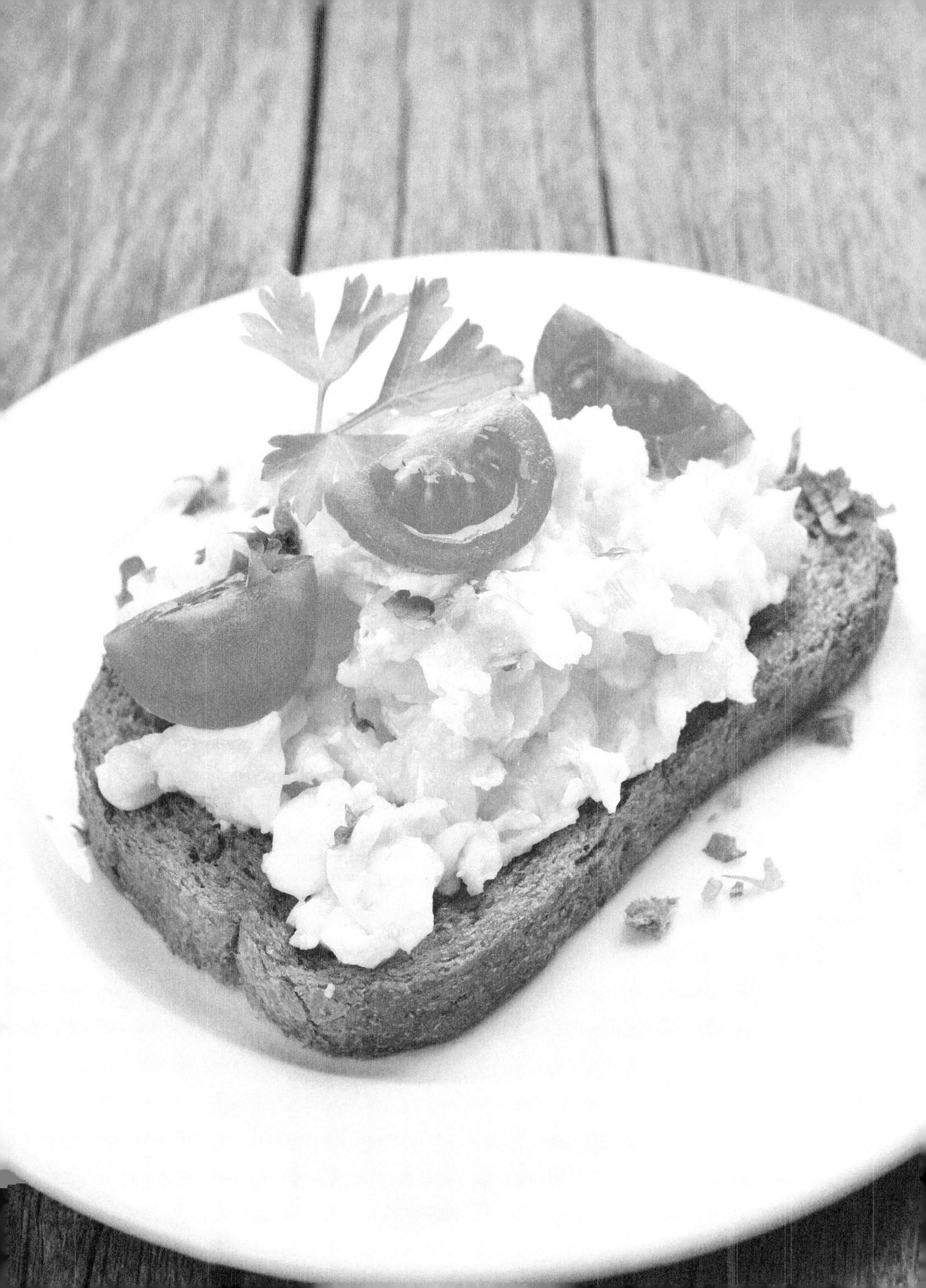

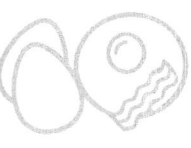

SPINACH AND EGG SCRAMBLE WITH RASPBERRIES

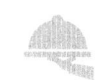

SERVINGS - 1

TIME - 10 min

 NUTRITIONAL VALUE

- Calories-296 cal
- Carbohydrates-21g
- Proteins-17.8g
- Fats-15.7g

 INGREDIENTS

- 1 tsp oil
- 1 cup baby spinach
- 2 large eggs
- Pinch of salt
- Pinch of ground pepper
- ½ cup raspberries
- 1 slice of a whole-grain wheat slice

 INSTRUCTIONS

1. Heat oil in the pan and add spinach leaves to it.
2. Crack eggs in a bowl and whisk them with slight seasonings of salt and pepper.
3. Add beaten egg mixture to the baby spinach leaves and fry eggs in it.
4. Put the scrambled egg over the toast and serve with raspberries.

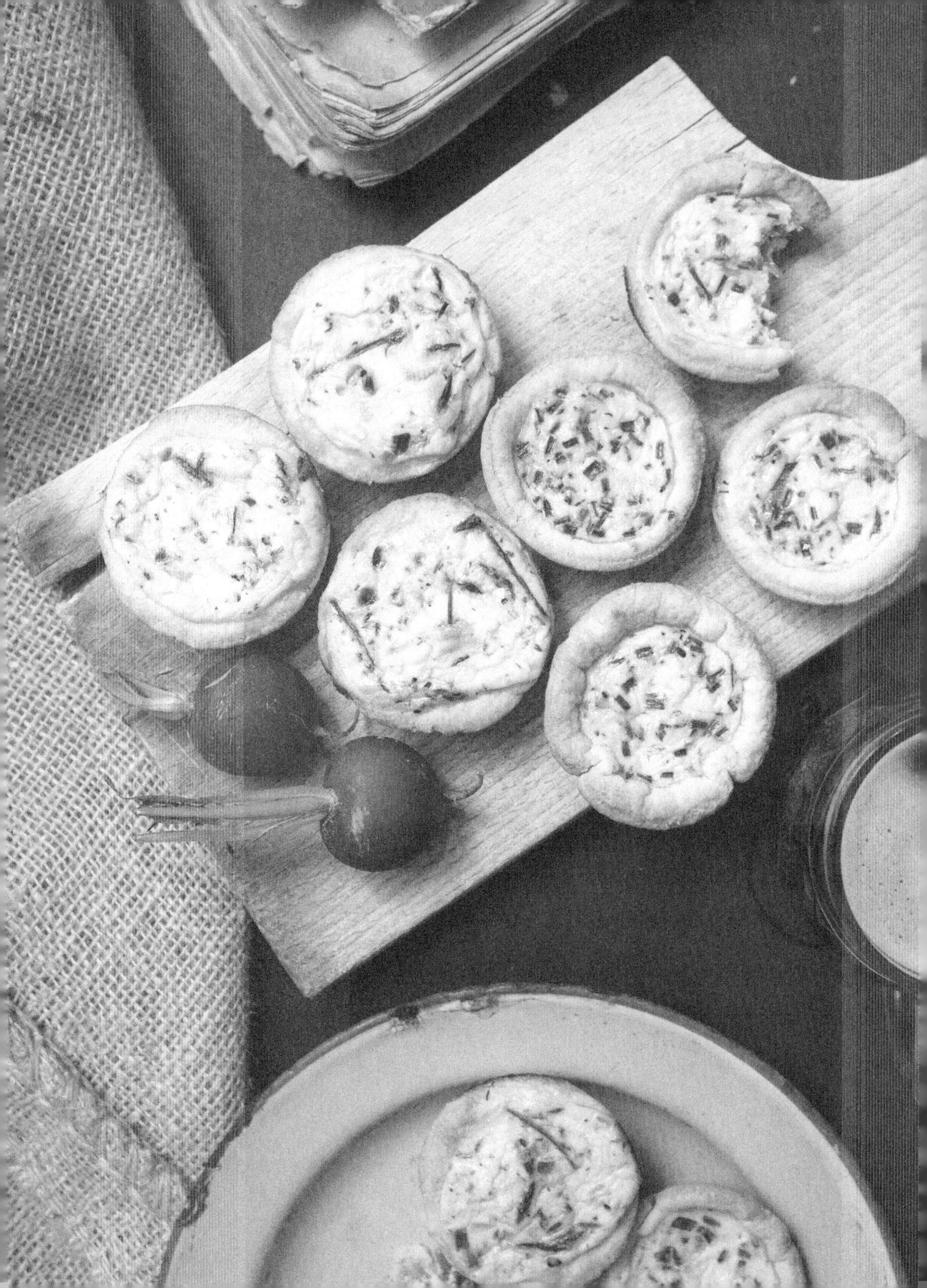

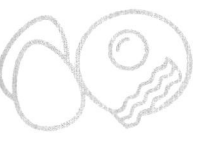

MINI FRITTATAS

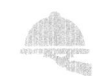

SERVINGS - 6

TIME - 20 min

 NUTRITIONAL VALUE

- Calories-234 kcal
- Carbohydrates-23g
- Proteins-34.5g
- Fats- 19g

 INGREDIENTS

- 6 large eggs
- ¼ cup milk
- 1 tsp salt
- ½ tsp black pepper
- ¼ cup artichokes
- 1/3 cup olives
- ¼ cup red peppers
- ½ cup tomatoes
- ½ cup cheese
- ¼ cup parsley leaves

 INSTRUCTIONS

1. In a blender crack eggs and add milk. You may whisk the mixture as well.
2. Pour the mixture into the greased muffin tray and don't forget to pre-heat your oven at 375 degrees Fahrenheit (190 degree Celsius).
3. Pour the mixture in such a way that only 3/4th of the cups get filled.
4. Sprinkle in some salt, pepper, chopped artichokes, halved olives, chopped red pepper, chopped tomatoes, shredded cheese, and chopped parsley leaves.
5. Put the tray into the oven for 12 to 15 minutes until all the things get baked.

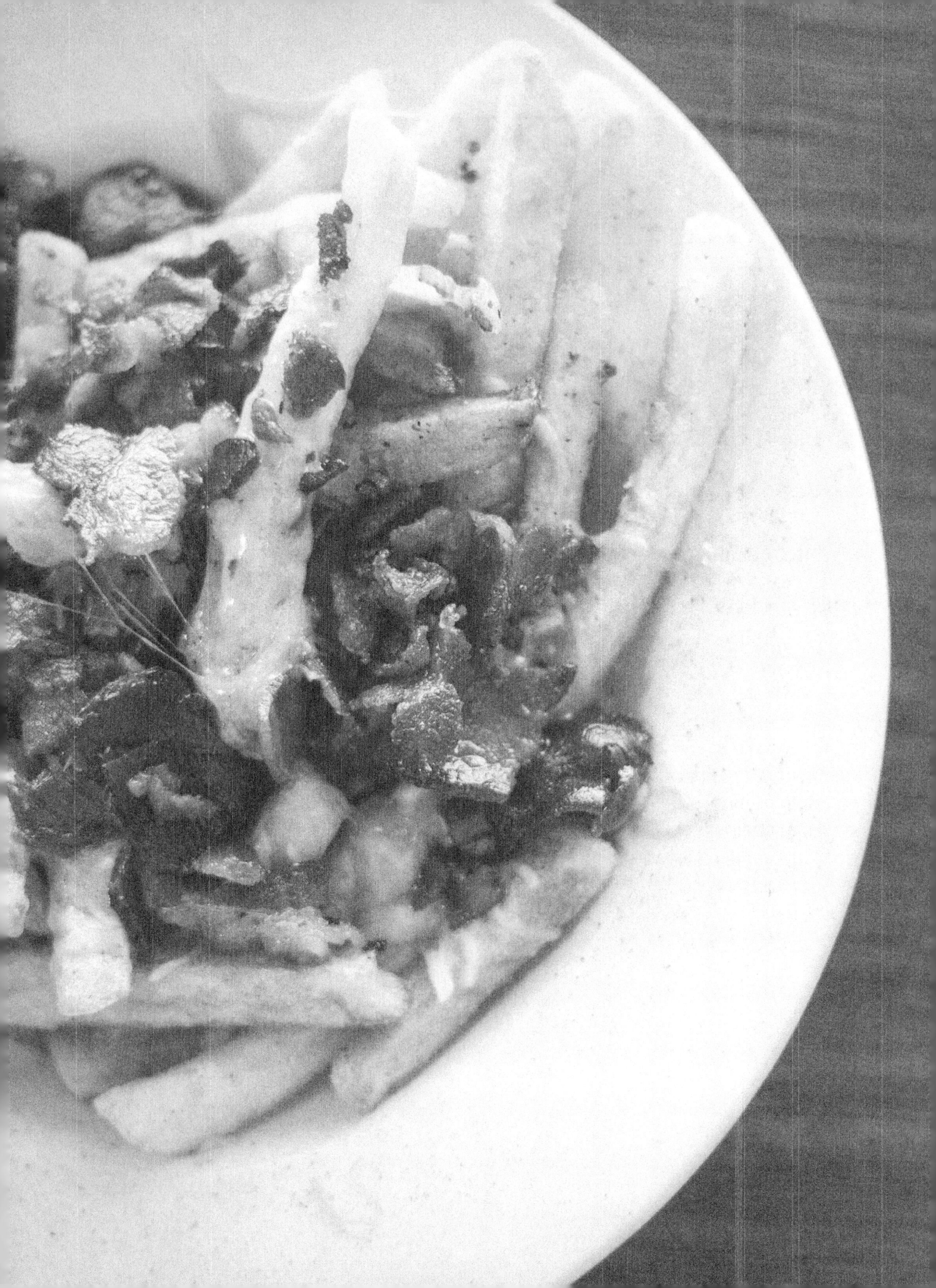

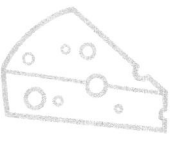

LOW CARB CHILI CHEESE FRIES

SERVINGS - 2

TIME - 30 min

NUTRITIONAL VALUE

- Calories- 637kcal
- Carbohydrates- 12.8g
- Proteins-26g
- Fats-51.3g

INGREDIENTS

Super simple chili
- 1 tbsp butter
- 1 small diced onion
- 1 large diced celery
- 2 minced garlic gloves
- 3 cups ground beef
- 1 diced red bell pepper
- 1 tsp chili powder
- 1 tsp ground cumin
- 1 tsp dried oregano
- 1 tin chopped tomatoes
- Salt as per taste
- Black as per taste
- 2 tbsp chopped cilantro
- 2 tbsp olive oil

Fries
- 3 medium turnips
- ½ tsp garlic powder
- ½ tsp paprika powder
- ½ tsp salt
- ¼ tsp black pepper
- ½ cup shredded cheese
- 4 tbsp sour cream
- 1 tbsp chopped cilantro
- 1 spring onion- green part only

INSTRUCTIONS

1. In a skillet add butter and sauté onions and celery for 2 minutes. After that add garlic and fry them.
2. Now add ground beef in it and fry for 5 minutes.
3. Then add chopped red bell pepper, spices, and tomatoes, and chopped cilantro. Mix everything and cook the beef mixture for 15 minutes.
4. Add some sour cream and fresh coriander into the super simple chili.
5. Cut the turnip into finger fries.
6. Place them onto a greased baking sheet. Bake the turnip strips for about 30-35 minutes until crispy.
7. To prepare your serving, add super simple chili onto the fries along with some shredded cheese and place back into the oven for 5 minutes.
8. At last chopped green onions, chopped coriander, and sour cream as a top garnish.

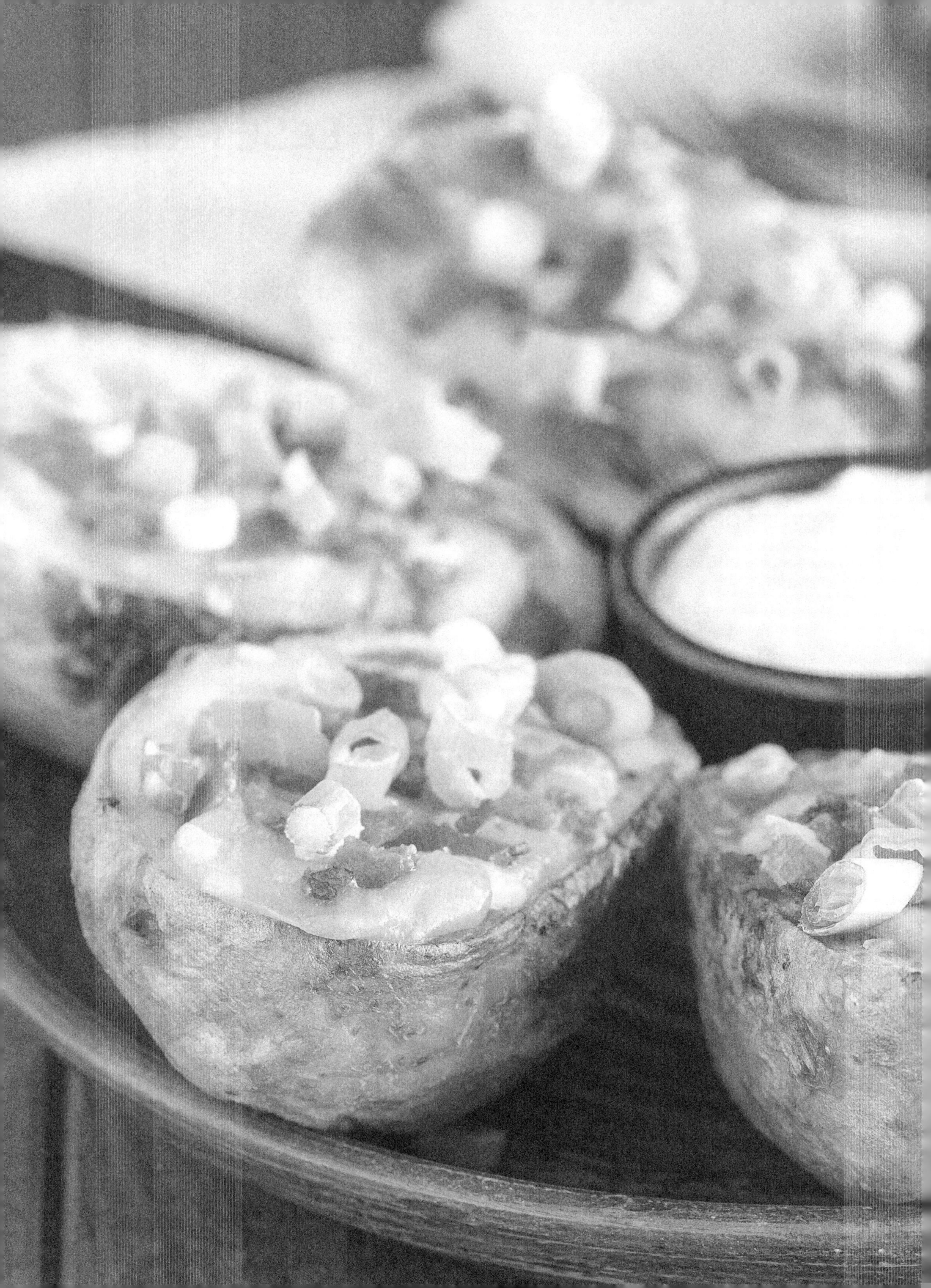

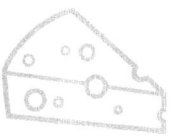

CHEESE AND BACON STUFFED MEAT PIES

SERVINGS - 3

TIME - 30 min

NUTRITIONAL VALUE

- Calories-737kcal
- Carbohydrates- 7.3g
- Proteins-44.1g
- Fats-59.3g

INGREDIENTS

Filling
- 2 cups ground beef
- ½ cup chopped bacon
- 1 chopped onion
- 1 tbsp coconut aminos
- 2 tbsp tomato sauce
- 1 cup beef stock
- ½ tsp xanthum gum

Pie crust
- 2 ½ cup shredded mozzarella cheese
- 1 tbsp cream cheese
- 1 ½ cup almond flour
- 2 large eggs
- 1 tsp onion powder
- 6 chunks of cheddar cheese

INSTRUCTIONS

1. In a skillet add butter, bacon, ground beef, and onion. Cook the constituents for a few minutes.
2. Add coconut aminos and beef stock and stir all the ingredients well. Also, put some xanthum gum and cook for a few more minutes.
3. Let the ground mixture cool down and preheat your oven at at 400 degree Fahrenheit (200 degrees Celsius).
4. To prepare crust to add all the ingredients to a separate bowl and mix them until a dough-like consistency is obtained. You may microwave your cheese for 30 seconds and then prepare the crust.
5. Take a muffin tray and grease all the muffin molds. Place the dough in such a way that the sides and the base of the muffin mold get covered with the dough layer.
6. Then fill the center with beef filling and place a small chunk of cheddar cheese in the center.
7. Cover your pie by making a last top layer of dough onto the beef filling and seal the contents.
8. Place the muffin tray in the oven for 10-15 minutes and enjoy.

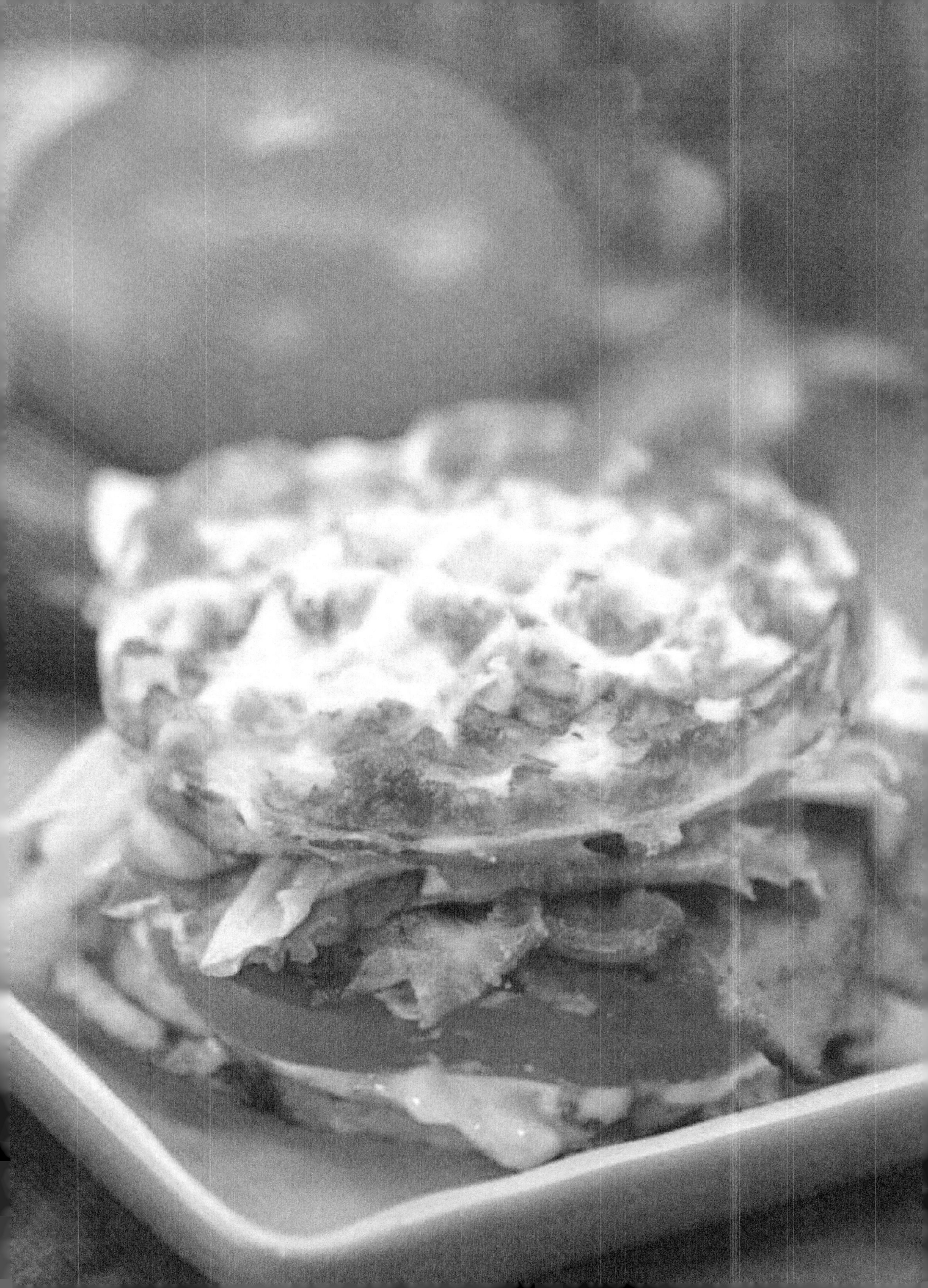

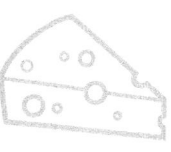

CHAFFLE SANDWICH

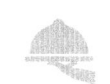

SERVINGS - 1

TIME - 20 min

NUTRITIONAL VALUE

- Calories- 458
- Carbohydrates- 3.5g
- Proteins-26.7g
- Fats-33.4g

INGREDIENTS

- ¾ cup shredded cheese
- 1 egg
- Salt as per taste
- Pepper as per taste
- 1 tsp hot sauce
- 1 tsp psyllium husk
- 4 slices bacon
- 4 slices ham
- 4 slices prosciutto
- 5-6 salami
- A bit mustard
- 1 tbsp mayonnaise

INSTRUCTIONS

1. Combine cheese, egg, salt, pepper, and psyllium husk in a bowl and place it in a greased waffle maker in 2 batches.
2. Cook it in a waffle maker for 2 to 3 minutes.
3. To prepare a sandwich, place all the remaining ingredients in between the cheese waffles and serve.

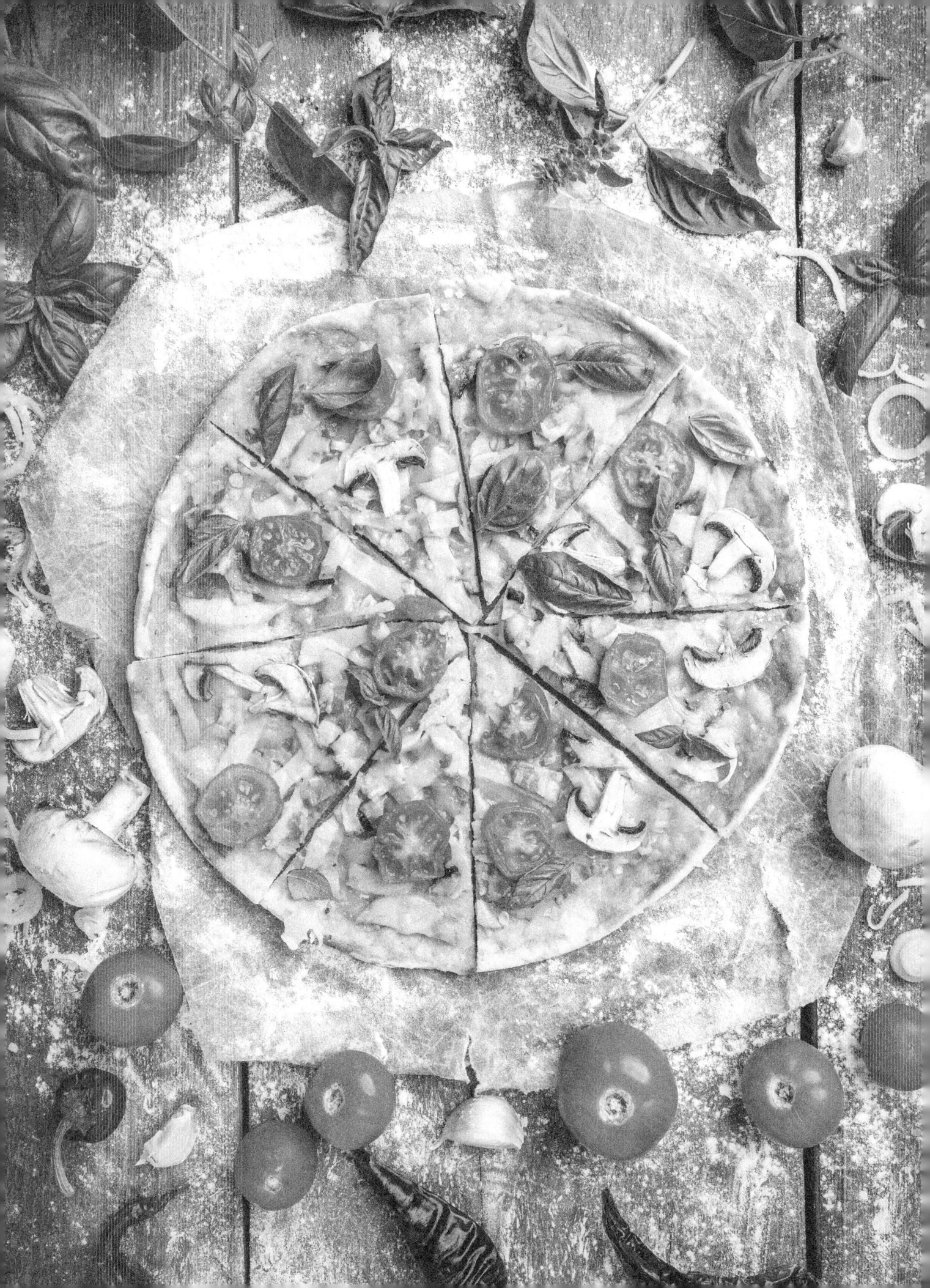

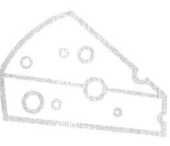

HEAD TRICOLORE PIZZA

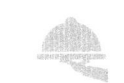

SERVINGS - 4

TIME - 40 min

 NUTRITIONAL VALUE

- Calories-619 kcal
- Carbohydrates-7.8g
- Proteins-49.1g
- Fats-43.3g

 INGREDIENTS

Head Fat head pizza base
- 1 ½ cup mozzarella
- 2 tbsp cream cheese
- 1 egg
- ½ tsp salt
- ¾ cup heaped almond flour

Pizza topping
- 1 1/8 cup chicken breast pieces
- ¼ tsp salt
- 1 pinch of black pepper
- 1 tsp olive oil
- ¼ cup sugar-free marinara sauce
- 1 cup sliced mozzarella
- 2 tbsp pesto
- 5 chopped sun-dried tomatoes

 INSTRUCTIONS

1. To prepare dough first add mozzarella slices and cream cheese into a bowl and microwave it for 30 seconds.
2. Take a large mixing bowl and add cream cheese mixture, egg, salt, pepper, and almond flour. Mix all the ingredients until a dough is formed.
3. Onto a baking sheet spread the dough and prick it with the help of a fork.
4. Cook chicken pieces by seasoning them and grilling them onto a griddle.
5. Spread marinara sauce onto the base and drizzle chicken pieces along with cheese pieces.
6. Bake the pizza in the preheated oven for 20 minutes.
7. Add some sun-dried tomatoes and pesto at the end. Serve with a sauce and enjoy!

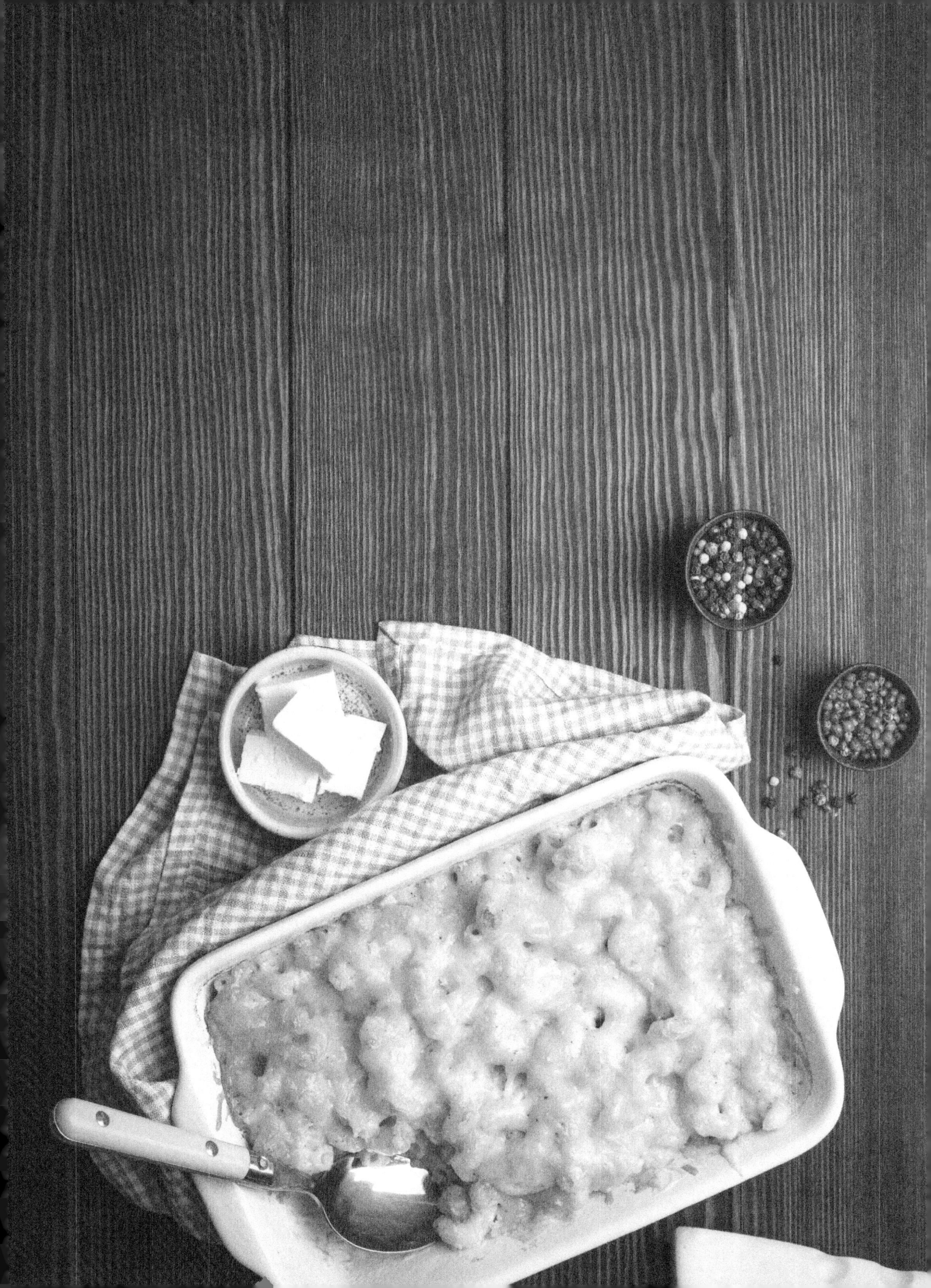

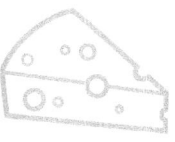

MEDITERRANEAN MACARONI AND CHEESE

SERVINGS - 6

TIME - 30 min

NUTRITIONAL VALUE

- Calories-405kcal
- Carbohydrates-55g
- Proteins-18g
- Fats-22g

INGREDIENTS

- 1 cup roasted diced tomatoes
- 1/3 cup chopped black olives
- 1 tbsp chopped fresh basil
- ½ tsp dried oregano
- Macaroni pasta
- 2 tbsp butter
- 2 tbsp olive oil
- 1/3 cup chopped red onion
- 1 minced large garlic clove
- 3 tbsp flour
- 2 cups almond milk
- Crumbled feta cheese
- Shredded mozzarella cheese
- Salt to taste
- Black pepper for taste

INSTRUCTIONS

1. Boil the pasta until it's soft and tender.
2. In a mixing bowl add tomatoes, olives, and basil and set it aside.
3. Take a saucepan and add butter into it. Now add onions and garlic and sauté them for 1 minute.
4. Then add flour and stir the contents well by using a whisk. Pour in some almond milk in batches after a few intervals with constant stirring. Sprinkle out some salt, pepper, and oregano into the saucepan.
5. Finally, add feta cheese along with some mozzarella cheese to thicken the sauce.
6. Assemble tomato salad over the drained pasta and drizzle over white sauce to enjoy the Mediterranean macaroni and cheese.

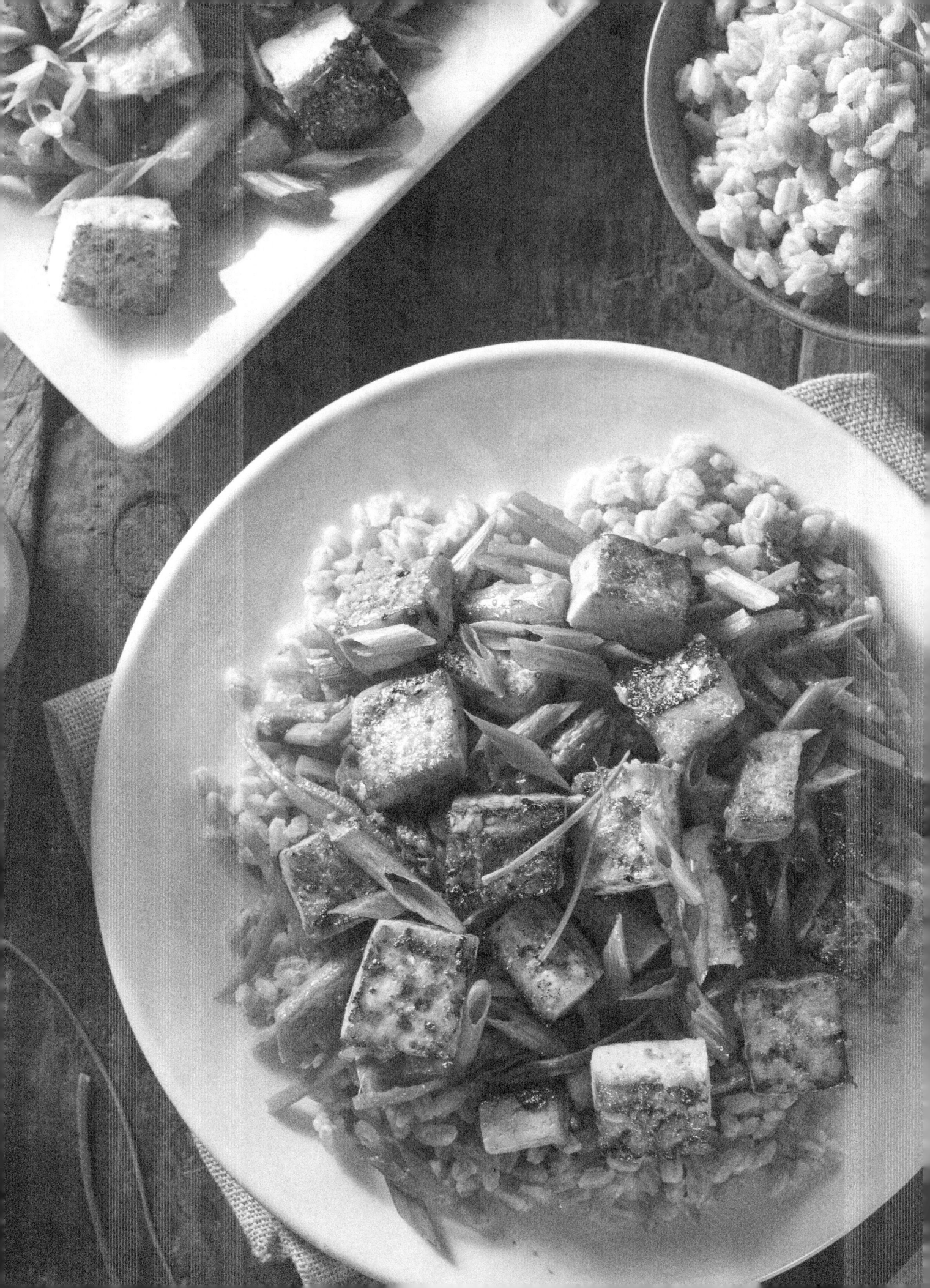

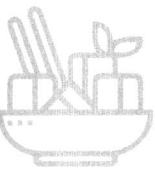

TOFU STIR FRY

SERVINGS - 4

TIME - 20 min

 NUTRITIONAL VALUE

- Calories-297 kcal
- Carbohydrates-12g
- Proteins-22g
- Fats-19g

 INGREDIENTS

- 1 1/2 cup tofu
- 1 tbsp vegetable oil
- 3 tbsp soy sauce
- 3 minced garlic cloves
- ¼ cup chopped green onions
- 2 tsp chili garlic paste
- 2 tsp grated ginger
- 1 cup baby spinach
- 2 tsp sesame leaves
- 2 tbsp roasted sesame seeds

 INSTRUCTIONS

1. Heat oil in a skillet and add tofu chunks into it. Heat the pieces until they are golden brown.
2. Add soy sauce along with ginger, garlic, green onions, chili garlic paste, and sesame oil.
3. After that add spinach leaves and sesame seeds. Stir fry everything.
4. Serve with cauliflower rice.

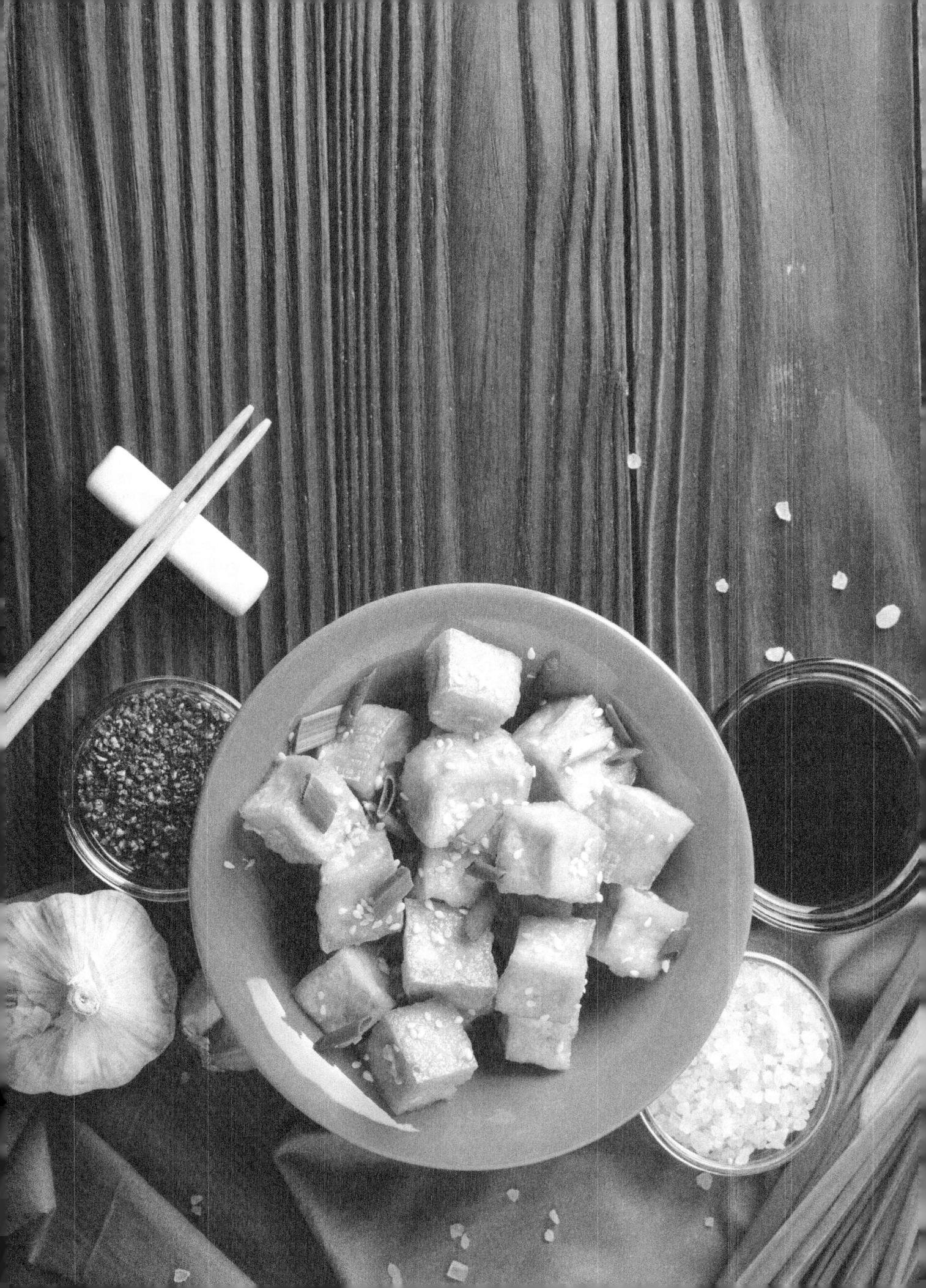

BAKED TOFU

SERVINGS - 2

TIME - 35 min

NUTRITIONAL VALUE

- Calories-298 kcal
- Carbohydrates-12g
- Proteins-19g
- Fats-22g

INGREDIENTS

- 1 cup cubed tofu chunks
- 2 tbsp olive oil
- 2 tbsp cornstarch
- ½ tsp salt
- ½ tsp pepper
- 1 tbsp of paprika

INSTRUCTIONS

1. Mix everything in a bowl and coat tofu pieces in cornstarch.
2. Pre-heat your oven at at 400 degrees Fahrenheit (200 degree Celsius) and place baking dish containing tofu in it for 30 minutes.
3. Serve them with a dip or sauce.

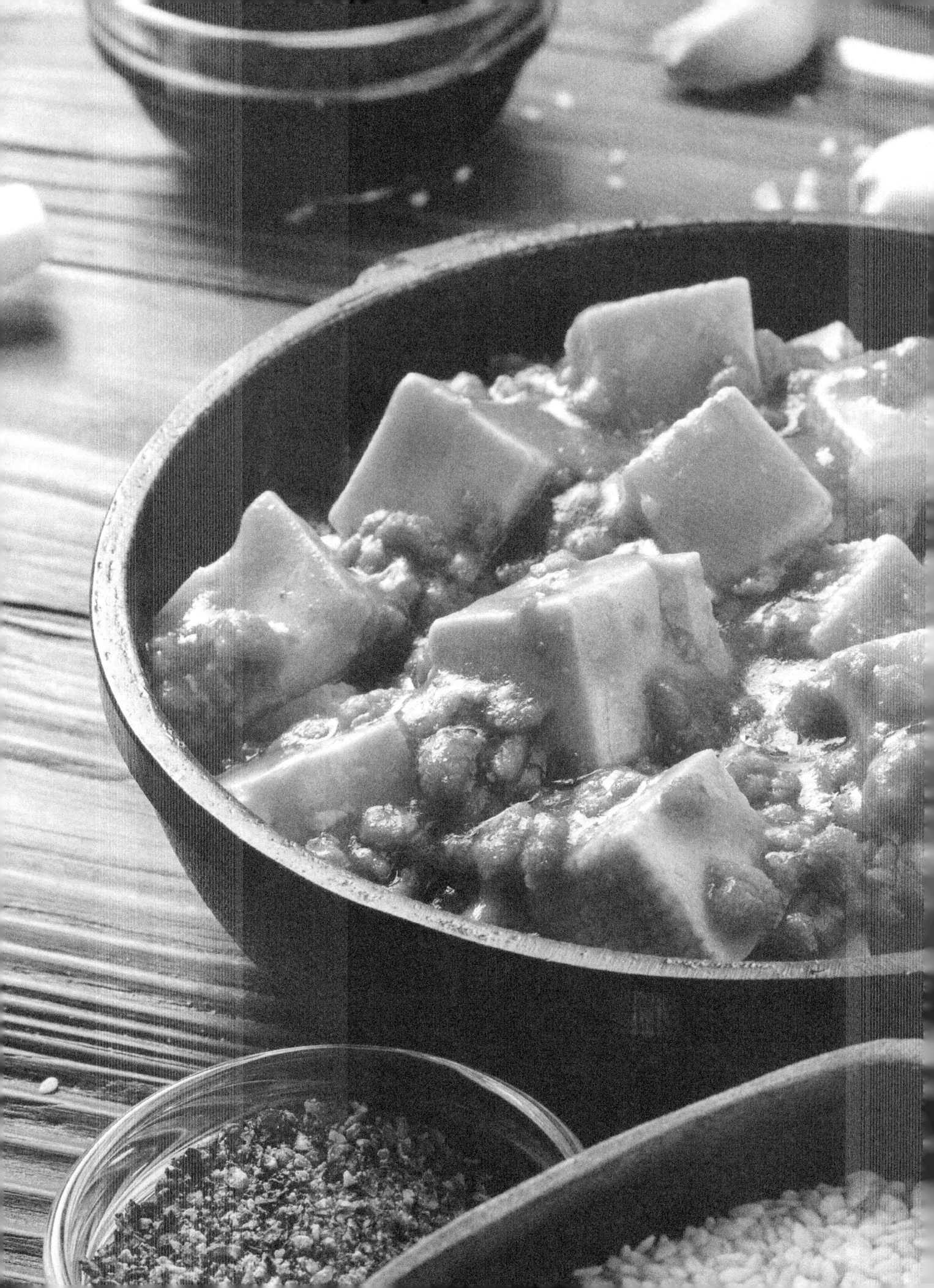

MAPO TOFU

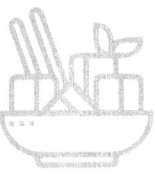

SERVINGS - 6

TIME - 35 min

NUTRITIONAL VALUE

- Calories-196 kcal
- Carbohydrates-5.7g
- Proteins-6.7g
- Fats-19g

INGREDIENTS

- 6 tbsp oil
- Tbsp. chili paste
- 2 tsp chopped black beans
- 1 tbsp chili flakes
- 2 tbsp cornstarch
- 2 tbsp water
- ¼ cup ground beef
- 1 tsp soy sauce
- ¼ cup scallions
- 1 ½ cup tofu

INSTRUCTIONS

1. In a mixing bowl add 5tbsp oil, chili paste, black beans, and chili flakes. Set it aside.
2. In another bowl add cornstarch and water and set it aside also.
3. In a pan add the remaining 1 tbsp oil and add ground beef. Cook beef for 10 minutes and transfer it into a small bowl.
4. In the same pan add scallions, soy sauce, and a bit of water. Add ground beef and tofu to the pan.
5. Then gradually add the cornstarch slurry and prepared paste mixture into the pan.
6. Cook the ingredients for 5 more minutes until everything combines well.

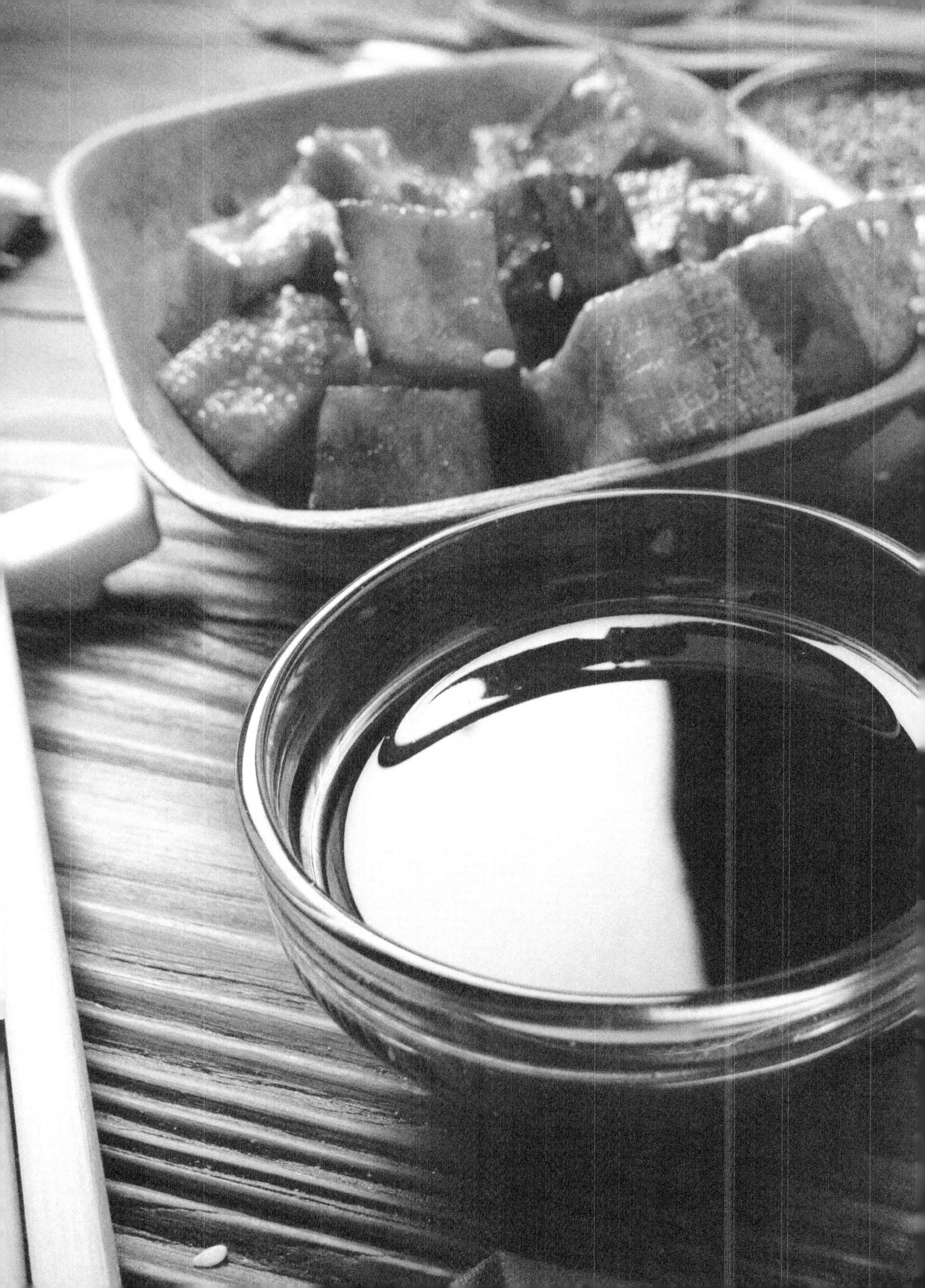

CRISPY MARINATED TOFU

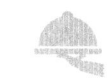

SERVINGS - 2

TIME - 35 min

NUTRITIONAL VALUE

- Calories-323 kcal
- Carbohydrates-2g
- Proteins-35g
- Fats-21g

INGREDIENTS

- 2tsp sesame oil
- 2 tsp soy sauce
- 2 tsp ginger garlic paste
- ½ tsp cayenne pepper
- 1 ½ cup tofu chunks

INSTRUCTIONS

1. Add all the ingredients into a mixing bowl and marinate the tofu chunks for 20 minutes.
2. Preheat your oven at 400 degrees and place marinated tofu chunks on the parchment paper in a baking sheet.
3. Bake tofu pieces for 30 minutes.

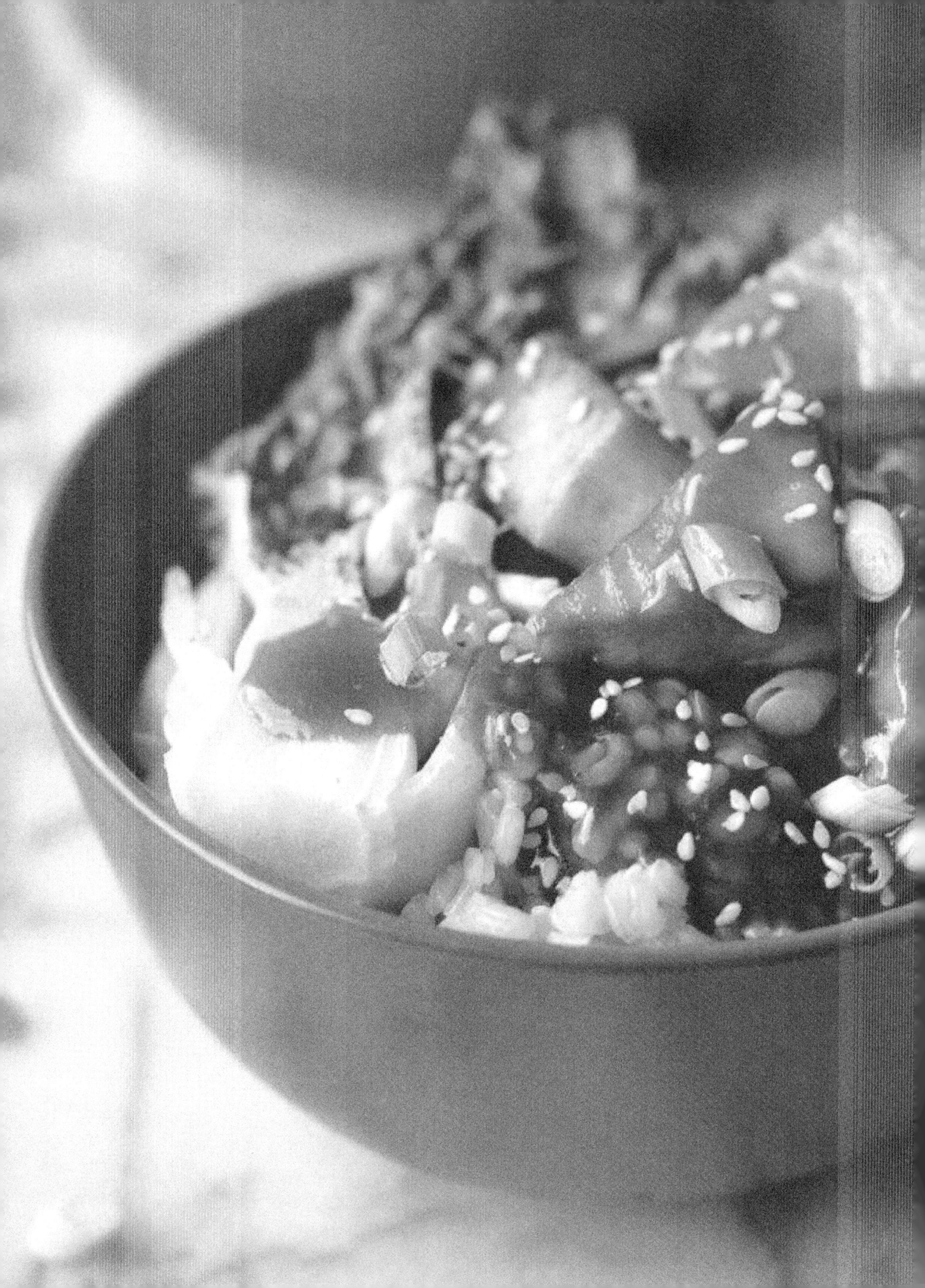

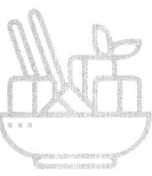

CRISPY BAKED TOFU WITH BOK CHOY

SERVINGS - 4

TIME - 30 min

 NUTRITIONAL VALUE

- Calories-209 kcal
- Carbohydrates-18g
- Proteins-12g
- Fats-18g

 INGREDIENTS

- 1 cup tofu
- ¼ cup plum sauce
- 3 tbsp ketchup
- 2 tbsp soy sauce
- 2 tsp oil
- 3 scallions
- 1 tsp minced garlic
- 4 baby bok choy
- ¼ cup water
- 1 tsp roasted sesame seeds

 INSTRUCTIONS

1. In a small mixing bowl, whisk plum sauce, garlic, ketchup, and soy sauce together.
2. Heat oil in a large skillet and add tofu in a single layer.
3. Add mixed sauces onto the tofu and cook for few minutes.
4. Also, add sesame seeds along with scallions into it and cook for 5 more minutes.
5. At the end serve with bok choy.

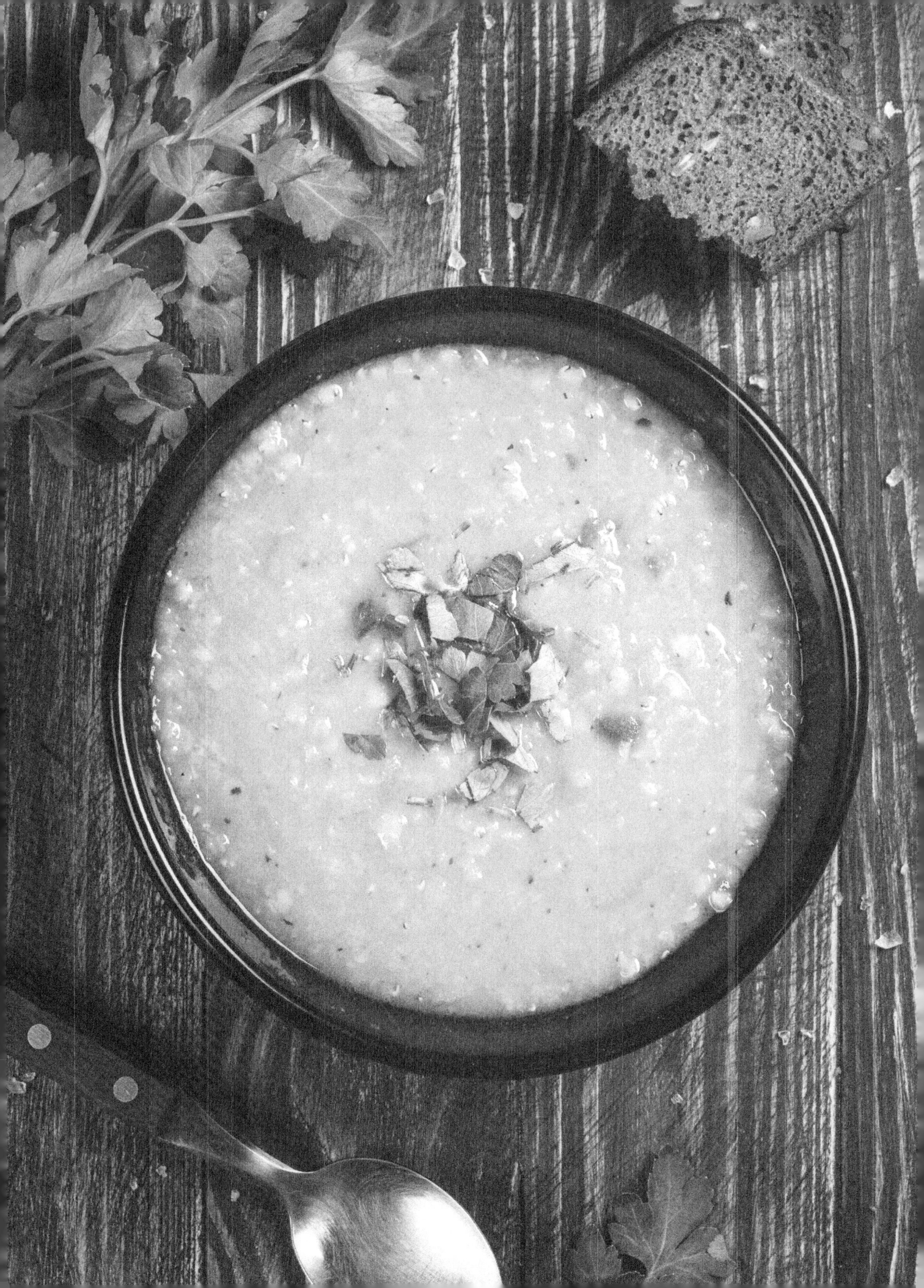

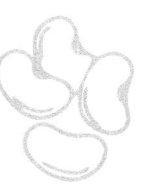

SPICED CARROT AND LENTIL SOUP

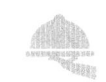

SERVINGS - 4

TIME - 25 min

NUTRITIONAL VALUE

- Calories-238 kcal
- Carbohydrates-34g
- Proteins-11g
- Fats-7g

INGREDIENTS

- 2 tsp cumin seeds
- 1 pinch chili flakes
- 2 tsp olive oil
- 2 cups grated carrots
- ½ cup split red lentils
- 4 cups vegetable stock
- ½ cup coconut milk

INSTRUCTIONS

1. Crackle cumin seeds and chili flakes in a pan on medium flame.
2. Pour in some olive oil, carrots, lentils, vegetable stock, coconut milk and bring the mixture to boil
3. Simmer the contents for 15 minutes until lentils are fully cooked and swollen.
4. Blitz the contents in a food processor to acquire a smooth consistency.

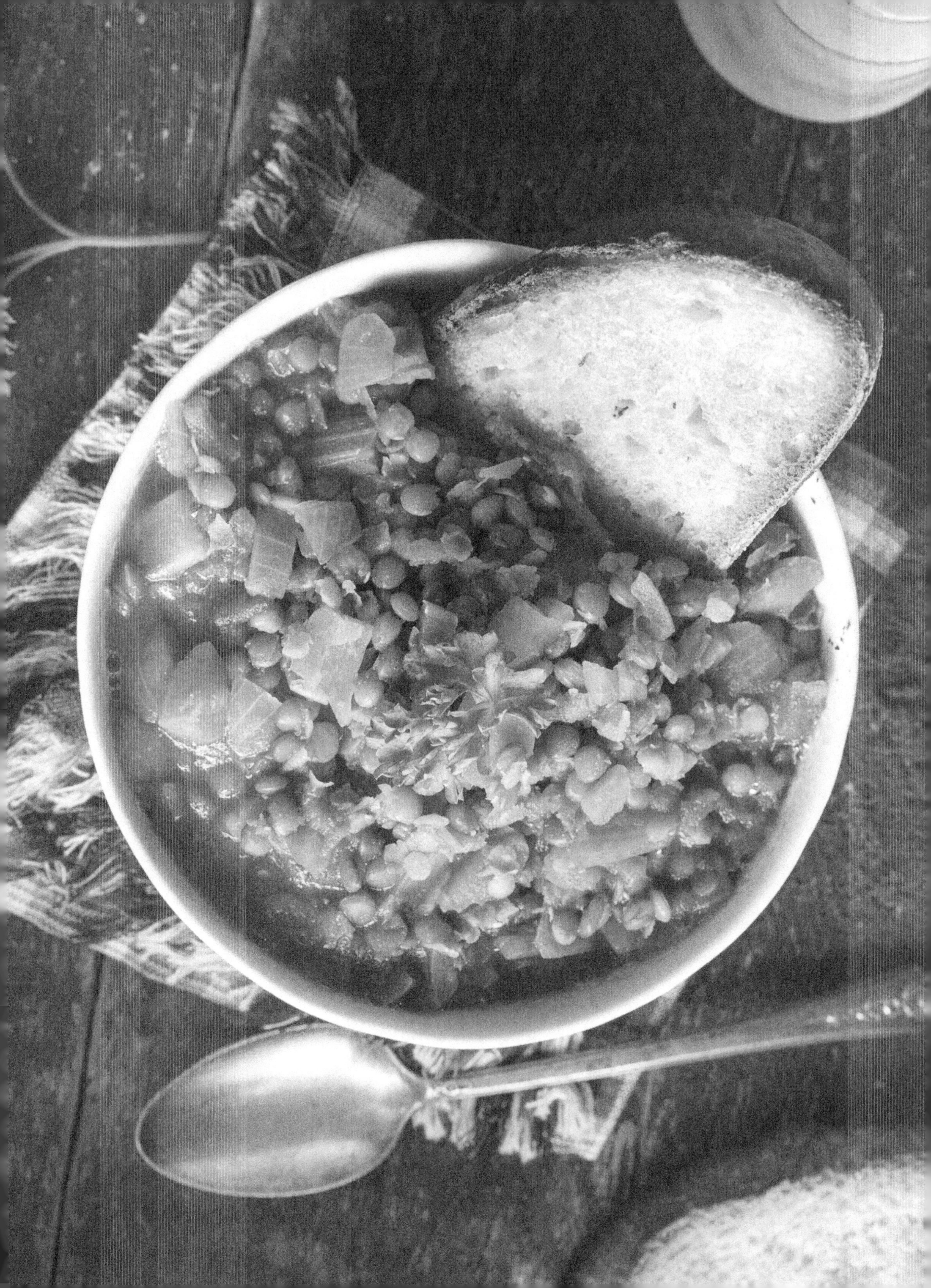

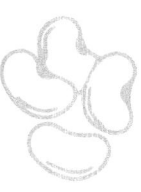

MEDITERRANEAN LENTIL SOUP

SERVINGS - 3

TIME - 20 mins

NUTRITIONAL VALUE

- Calories-464kcal
- Carbohydrates-63.1g
- Proteins-48.8g
- Fats-12.1g

INGREDIENTS

- 2 tbsp olive oil
- 1 cup chopped onions
- 1 cup chopped carrots
- 3 minced garlic clove
- 2 tbsp tomato paste
- 4 cups vegetable broth
- 1 cup water
- 1 cup cannellini beans
- 1 cup mixed lentils
- ½ cup chopped tomatoes
- ¾ tsp salt
- ½ tsp ground pepper
- 1 tbsp chopped fresh dill
- 1 tsp vinegar

INSTRUCTIONS

1. Take a large pan and add oil, onions, and garlic into it. Sauté them for 2 minutes.
2. After that add carrots with some tomato paste until carrots are soft and tender.
3. Add broth, water, lentils, cannellini beans, tomatoes, salt, and pepper to the same pan and cook it until things get well combined.
4. Serve the hot soup with vinegar and dill sprinkled on top.

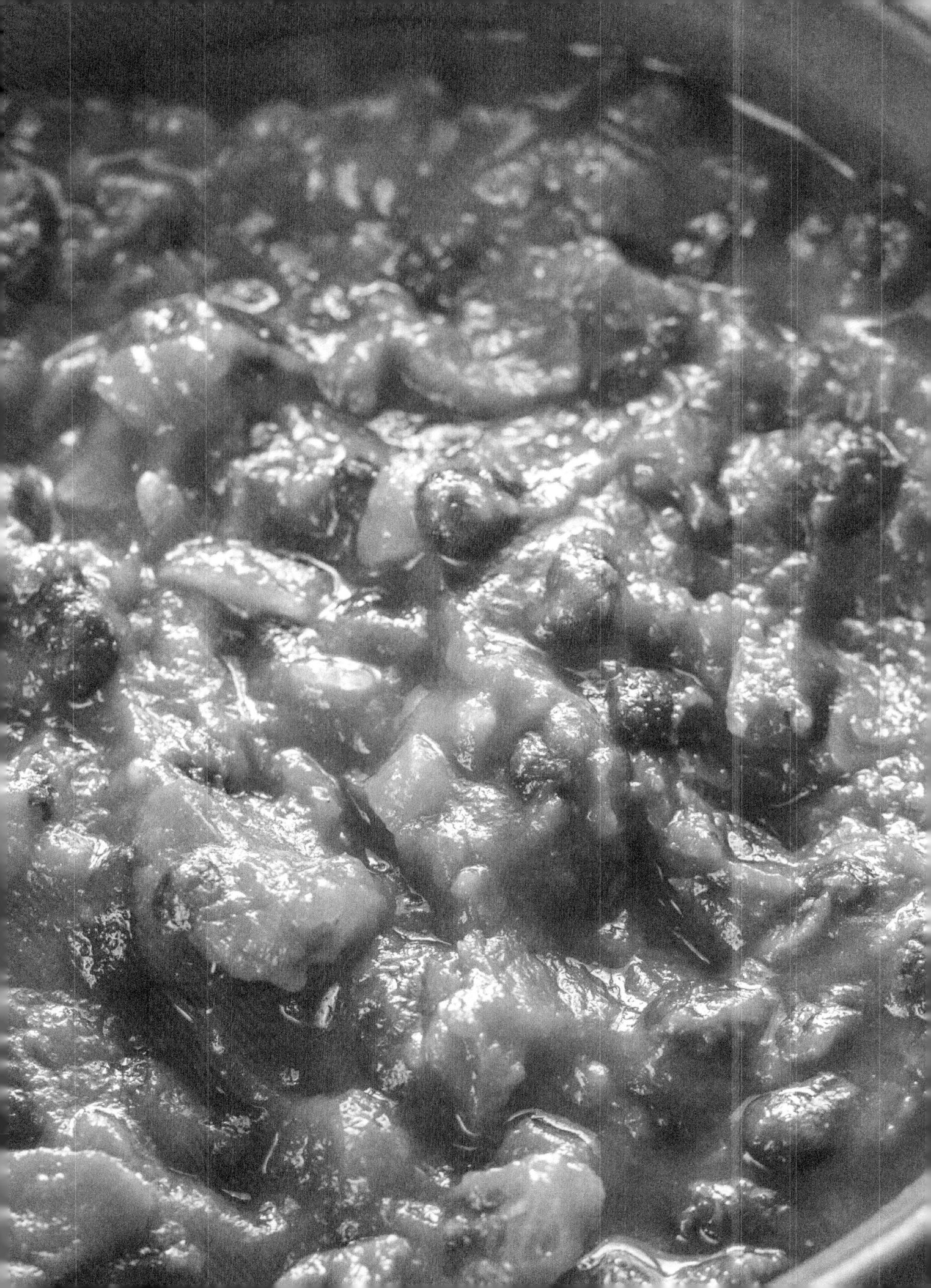

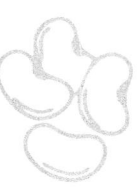

BLACK BEAN MUSHROOM CHILI

SERVINGS - 10

TIME - 5 Hrs

 NUTRITIONAL VALUE

- Calories-299 cal
- Carbohydrates-39g
- Proteins-18g
- Fats-10g

 INGREDIENTS

- 2 cups black beans
- 1 tbsp olive oil
- ¼ cup mustard seeds
- 2 tbsp chili powder
- 1 ½ tsp cumin seeds
- ½ tsp cardamom seeds
- 2 chopped onions
- 1 cup mushrooms
- ½ cup tomato paste
- ¼ cup water
- 5 cups mushroom broth
- 1 tbsp chipotle peppers in adobo sauce
- 1 1/4 cup grated cheese
- ½ cup cilantro

 INSTRUCTIONS

1. Soak beans overnight and boil them in water until they are fully cooked.
2. In a pot add oil, onions, mustard seeds, chili powder, cumin, and cardamom. Heat them until they start to crackle.
3. After that add mushrooms, tomatoes, and water.
4. Cook for a few minutes until everything becomes soft and then add broth along with some chipotles.
5. In a slow cooker add beans and prepared vegetable and bean mixture. Cover the lid and cook the contents on low heat for 3 hours.
6. Garnish your bowl with cilantro and serve.

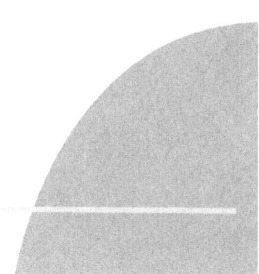

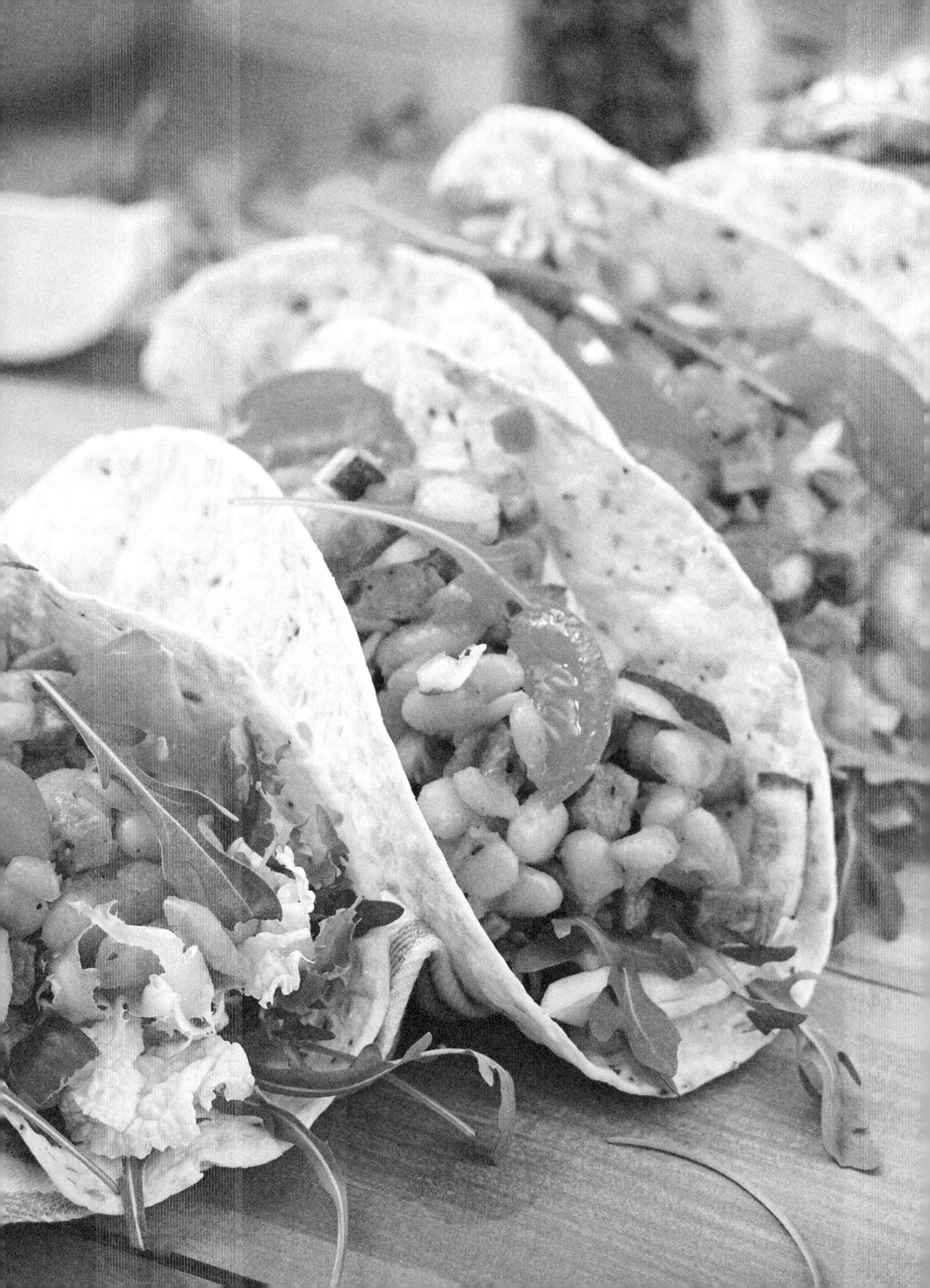

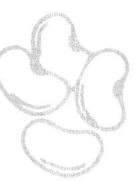

BLACK BEAN TACOS

SERVINGS - 2

TIME - 15 min

 NUTRITIONAL VALUE

- Calories-239kcal
- Carbohydrates-30.1g
- Proteins-12.8g
- Fats-14g

 INGREDIENTS

- 1 cup boiled black beans
- 4 taco shells
- 1 cup shredded lettuce
- 1/3 cup shredded cheese
- ¼ cup sour cream
- ¼ cup salsa

 INSTRUCTIONS

1. Mash cooked black beans with a masher and transfer the crumbled mixture to a taco shell.
2. Add some shredded lettuce, cheese along with some salsa and sour cream.
3. Wrap up taco shell and enjoy!

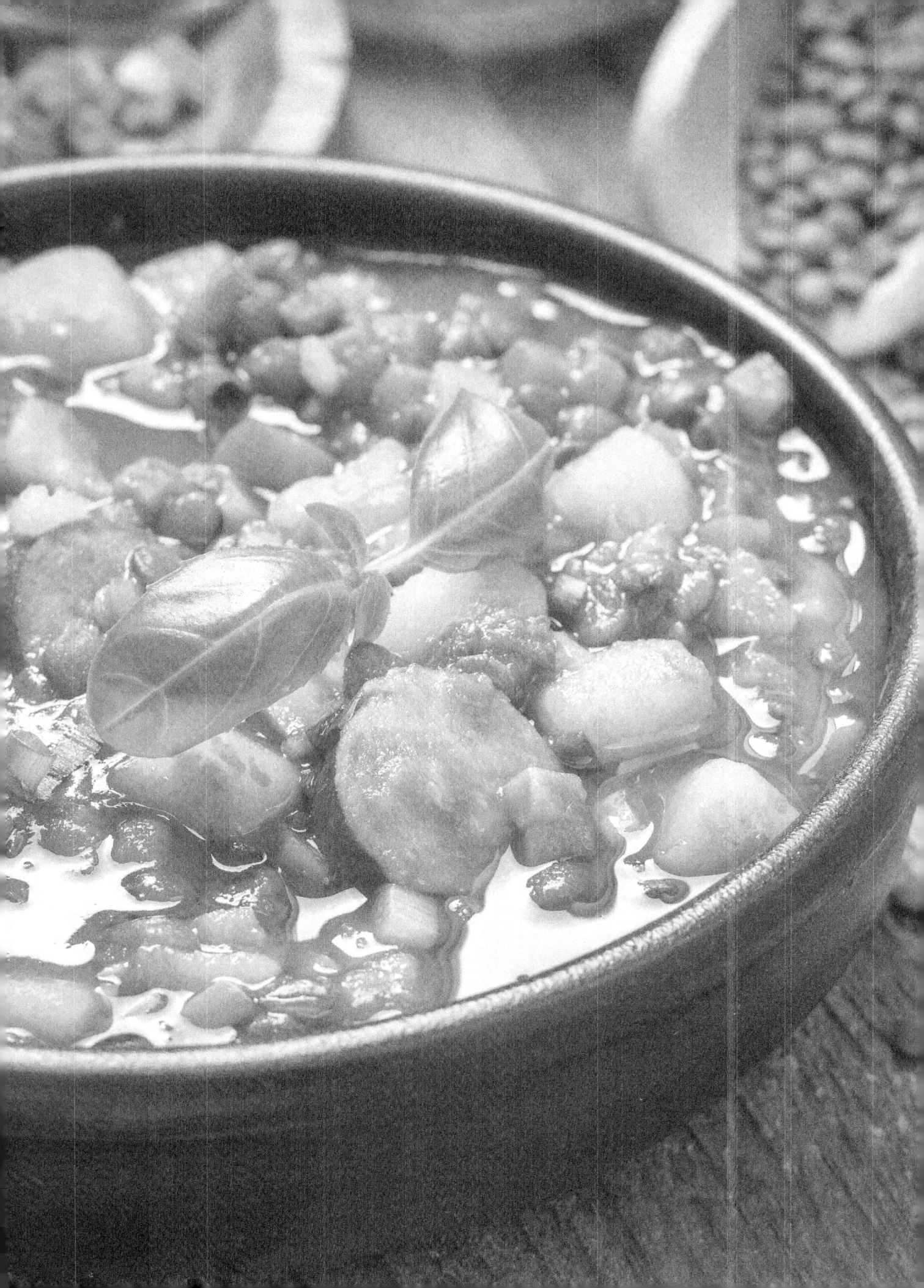

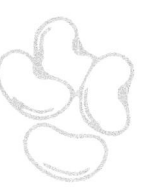

VEGAN LENTIL SOUP

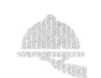

SERVINGS - 4

TIME - 40 min

NUTRITIONAL VALUE

- Calories-356kcal
- Carbohydrates-34g
- Proteins-56g
- Fats-24g

INGREDIENTS

- 2 tbsp olive oil
- 1 cup chopped onion
- 1 tbsp minced garlic
- 2 tsp turmeric
- 1 tsp ground ginger
- ½ tsp ground cumin
- 4 cups vegetable broth
- 1 cup dry lentil
- 1 cup chickpeas
- 1 cup chopped spinach
- 1 cup green beans
- 1 tbsp lemon juice
- 1 tsp red pepper
- Cilantro for garnishing

INSTRUCTIONS

1. Take a pot and add oil along with some chopped onions.
2. Then add garlic along with ginger and then add turmeric, cumin, and soaked chickpeas, dry lentil, and green beans.
3. Cook until the oil separates out and then add vegetable broth and chopped spinach.
4. Cook for half an hour and add lemon juice along with some seasoning at the end.
5. Simmer the contents for 20 minutes.
6. Garnish with cilantro leaves at the end.

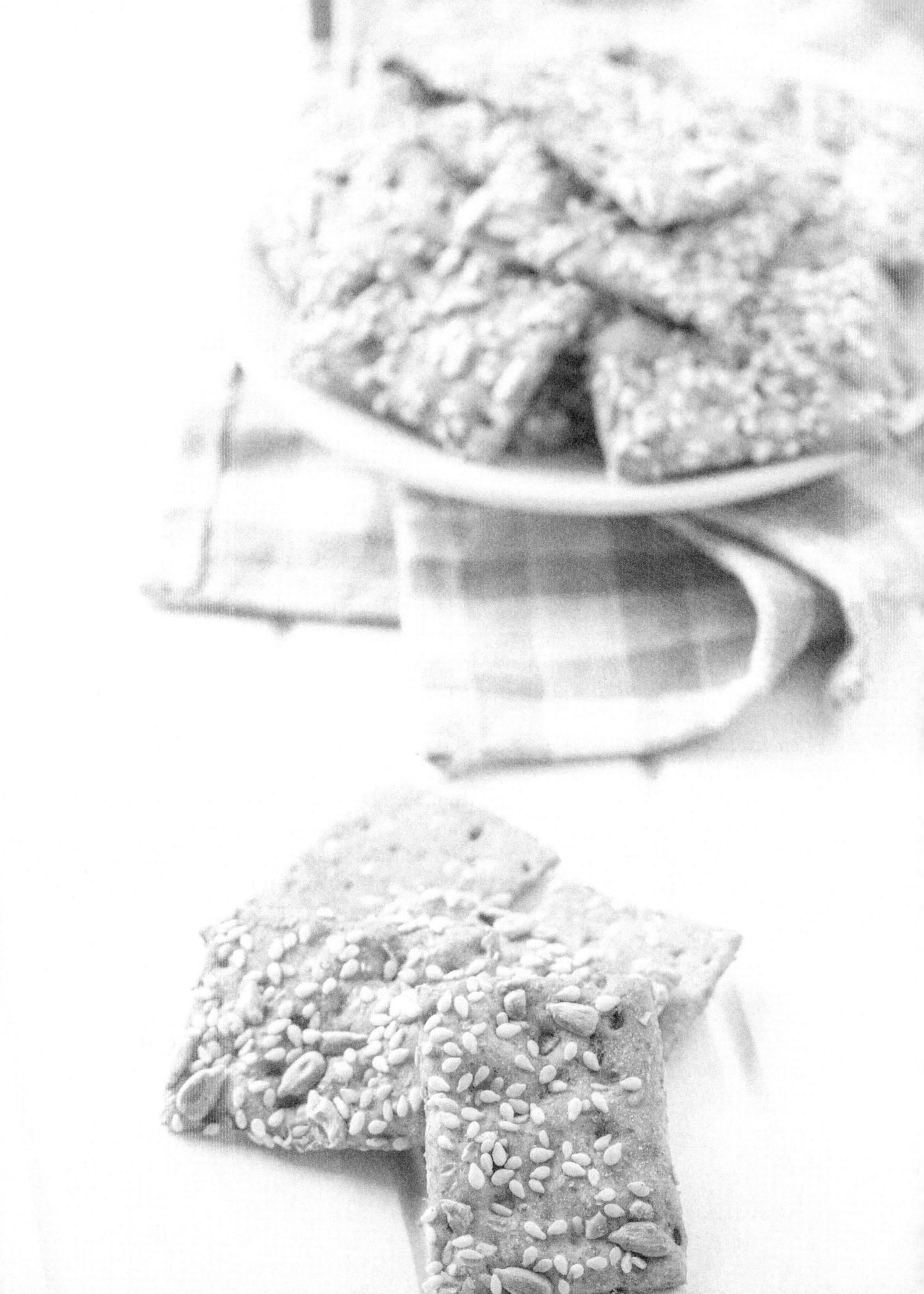

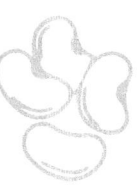

SEED CRACKERS

SERVINGS - 6

TIME - 40 min

 NUTRITIONAL VALUE

- Calories-60kcal
- Carbohydrates-1g
- Proteins-2g
- Fats-6g

 INGREDIENTS

- 1/3 cup almond flour
- 1/3 cup sunflower seeds
- 1/3 cup pumpkin seeds
- 1/3 cup chia seeds
- 1/3 cup sesame seeds
- 1 tbsp ground psyllium husk powder
- 1 tsp salt
- ¼ cup melted coconut oil
- 1 cup boiling water

 INSTRUCTIONS

1. Mix all the ingredients in a bowl and add melted oil and water to it.
2. Mix the contents until a gel-like consistency is obtained.
3. Spread the mixture onto a baking tray with parchment paper-lined below it. Also, place a layer of parchment paper above it.
4. Cook the cracker mixture for 30 minutes and serve the crunch explosion.

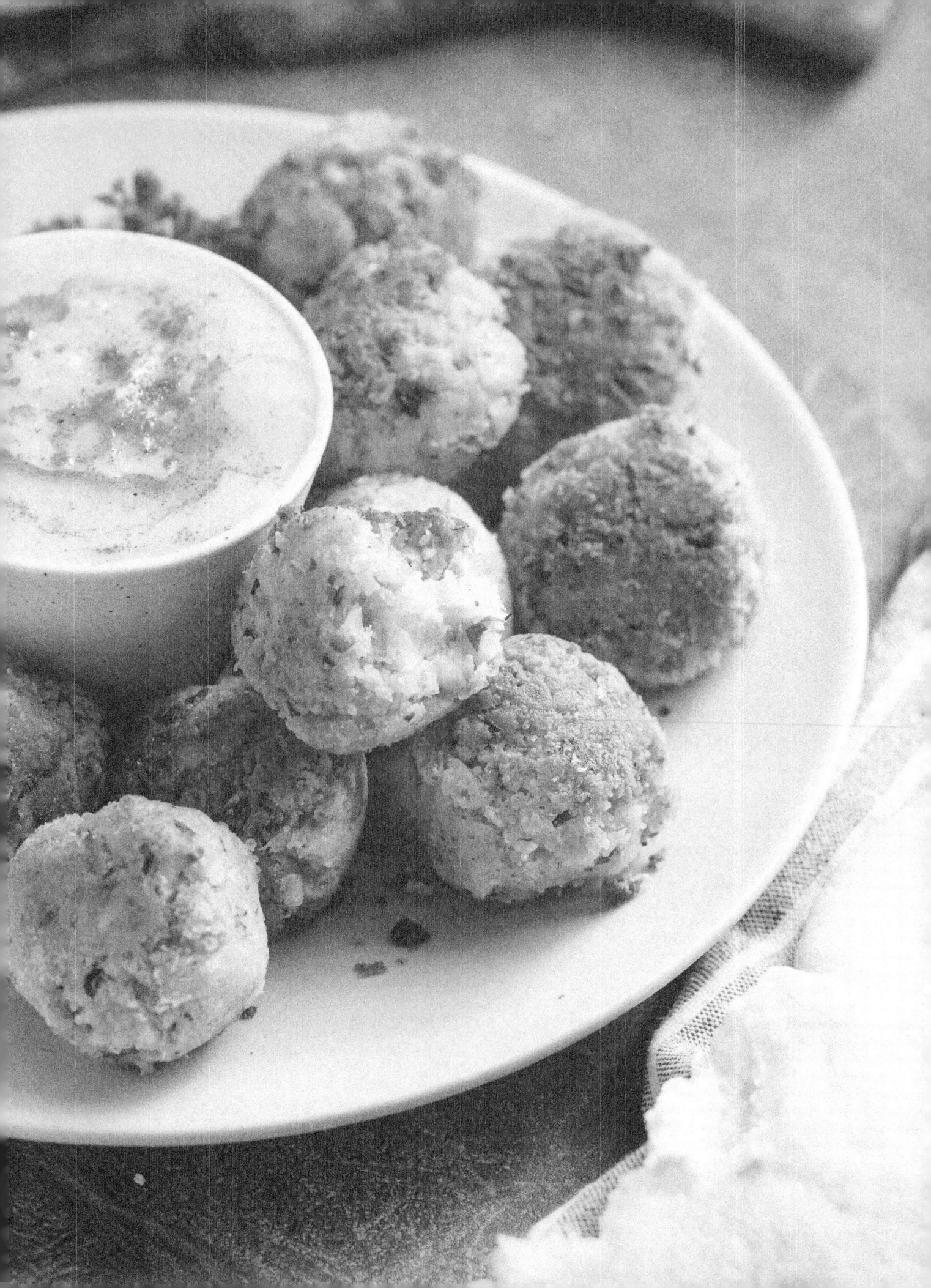

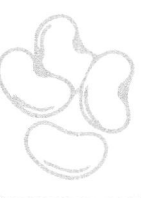

FALAFEL

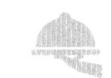

SERVINGS - 12

TIME - 50 min

 NUTRITIONAL VALUE

- Calories-178 kcal
- Carbohydrates-25g
- Proteins-12g
- Fats-4g

 INGREDIENTS

- 2 cups cooked chickpeas
- ½ tsp baking soda
- ¾ cup chopped fresh cilantro leaves
- 7-8 minced garlic
- 1 tbsp ground black pepper
- ½ cup chopped fresh dill
- 1 tbsp ground cumin
- 1 tbsp ground coriander
- 1 small diced onion
- 2 tbsp roasted sesame seeds
- 1 cup chopped fresh parsley leaves
- Salt to taste
- Oil for frying
- 3 tbsp tahini sauce
- 12 Pita pockets
- 1 cup diced cucumber
- 1 cup diced tomatoes
- 1 cup pickles

 INSTRUCTIONS

1. In a food processor add chickpeas, parsley, dill, cilantro, onions, salt, black pepper, ground cumin, and ground coriander along with garlic cloves.
2. Run the processor until a smooth mixture is obtained.
3. Add baking powder and sesame seeds to the falafel mixture.
4. Make 24 falafel patties out of the mixture
5. Heat the oil for frying purposes
6. Fry the patties in the oil until they are crispy
7. Assemble falafel patties inside the pita bread lined by tahini sauce, some pickles, tomatoes, and cucumber pieces.

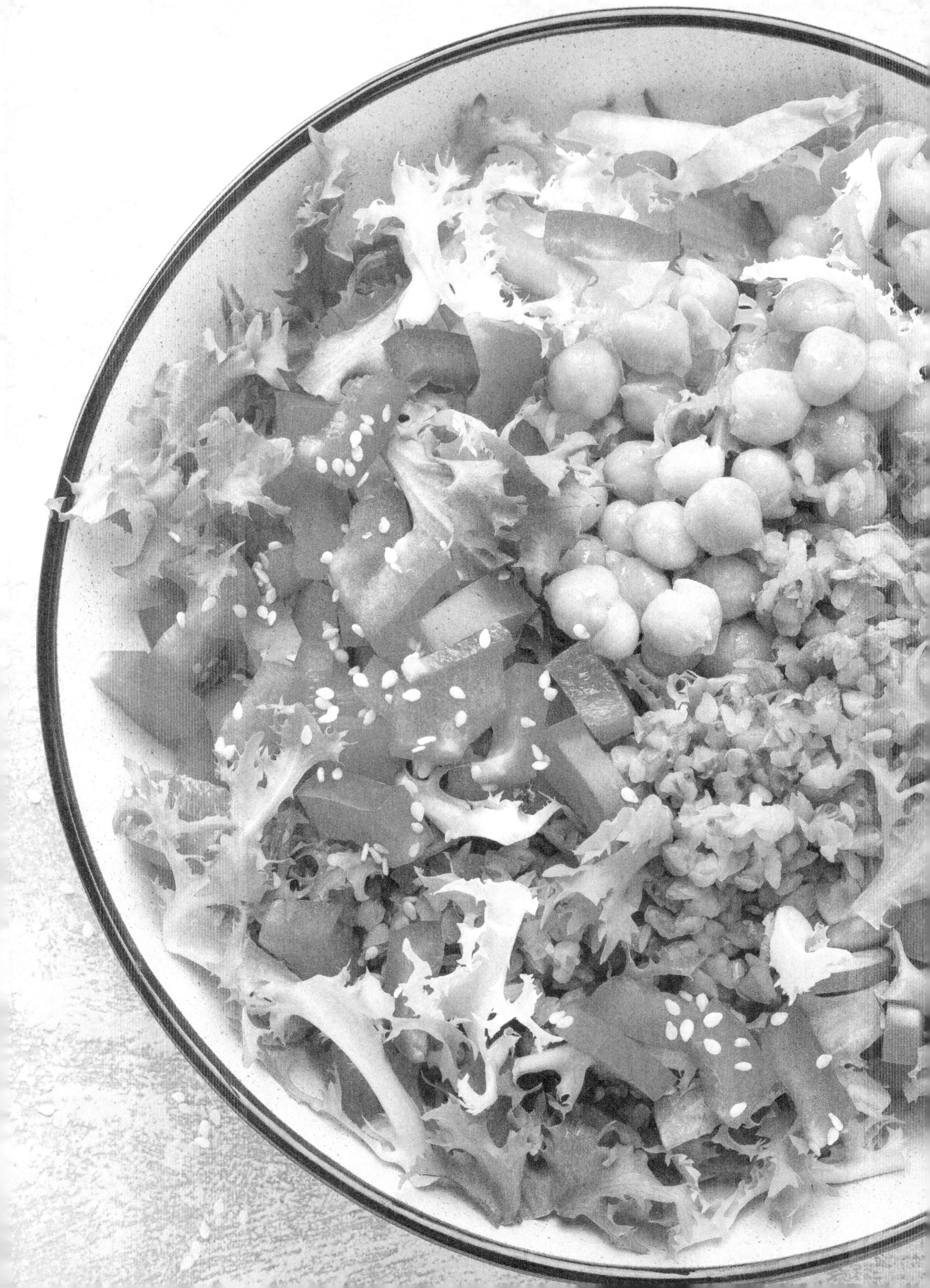

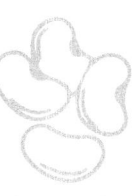

VEGAN CHICKPEA BOWL

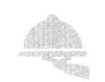

SERVINGS - 3

TIME - 20 min

 NUTRITIONAL VALUE

- Calories- 1016kcal
- Carbohydrates- 129.5g
- Proteins-32.9g
- Fats-49g

 INGREDIENTS

- 1 diced sweet potato
- 3 tbsp olive oil
- ½ tsp salt
- ½ tsp ground pepper
- 2 tbsp tahini
- 2 tbsp water
- 1 tbsp lemon juice
- 1 minced garlic clove
- 2 cups cooked quinoa
- 1 cup boiled chickpeas
- 1 diced avocado
- ¼ cup chopped parsley

 INSTRUCTIONS

1. In a pan add olive oil and toss sweet potatoes with some salt and pepper.
2. To prepare sauce, mix tahini, lemon juice, water, garlic, and salt. Whisk them well until a sauce-like consistency is obtained.
3. To prepare the serving bowl to add in cooked quinoa, avocado, and chickpeas. Then add some sweet potato pieces and drizzle over some sauce to complete the salad.

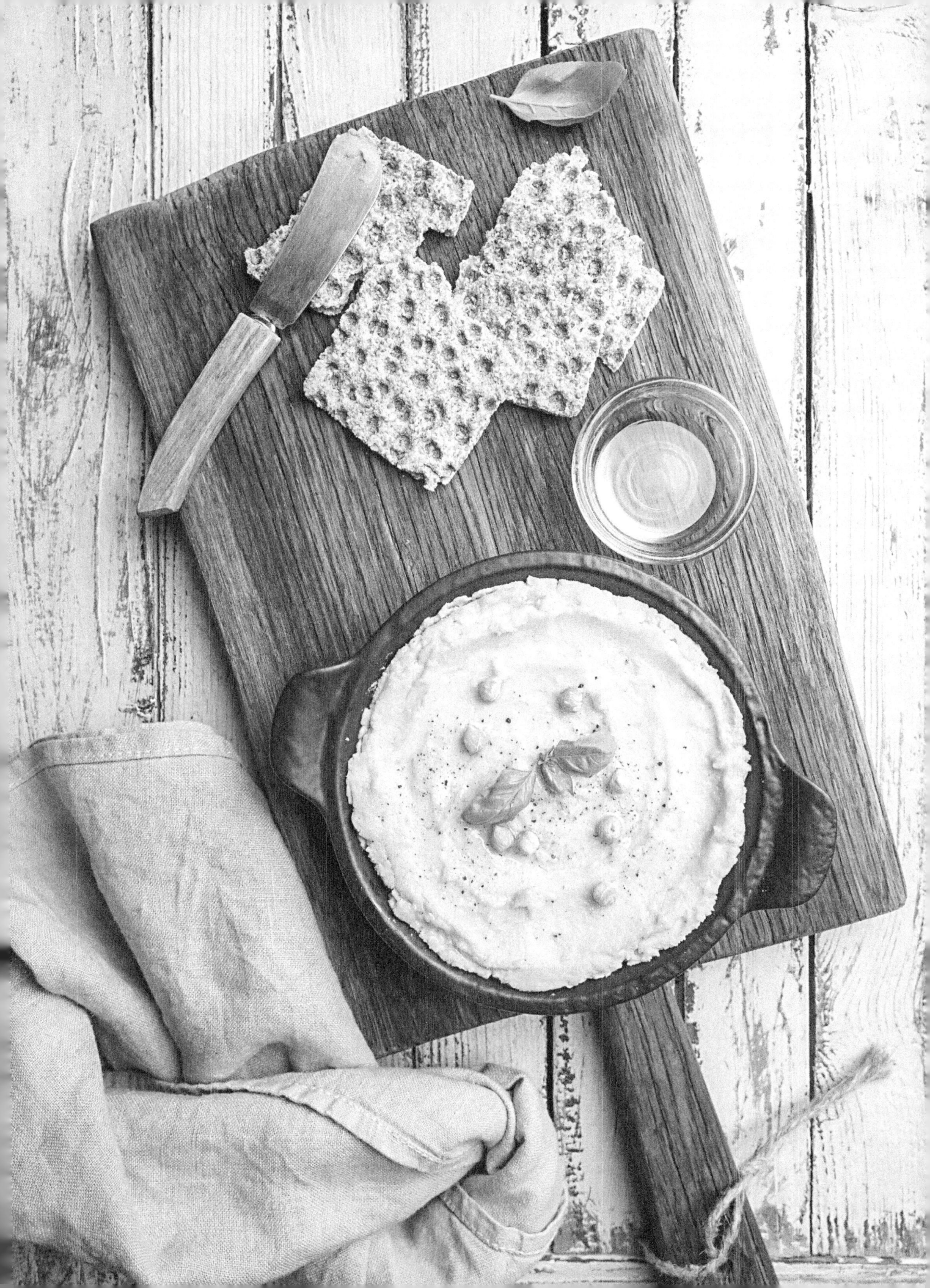

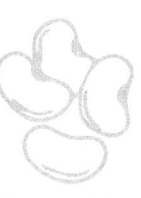

HEALTHY HUMMUS

SERVINGS - 4

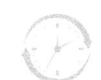

TIME - 30 min

NUTRITIONAL VALUE

- Calories-166 k cal
- Carbohydrates-14.3 g
- Proteins-7.9g
- Fats-9.6g

INGREDIENTS

- 3 quarts water
- 1 tsp baking soda
- ½ tsp salt
- ½ tsp black pepper
- 1/3 cup tahini sauce
- 1 cup chickpeas
- 2 tbsp lemon juice
- 2 minced garlic cloves
- ¼ tsp cumin

INSTRUCTIONS

1. Boil chickpeas by adding baking soda and salt to the water.
2. Transfer boiled chickpeas, tahini, garlic cloves, lemon juice, cumin, and ½ cup of water in the food processor.
3. Season the mixture well and run the blender to make a smooth paste.

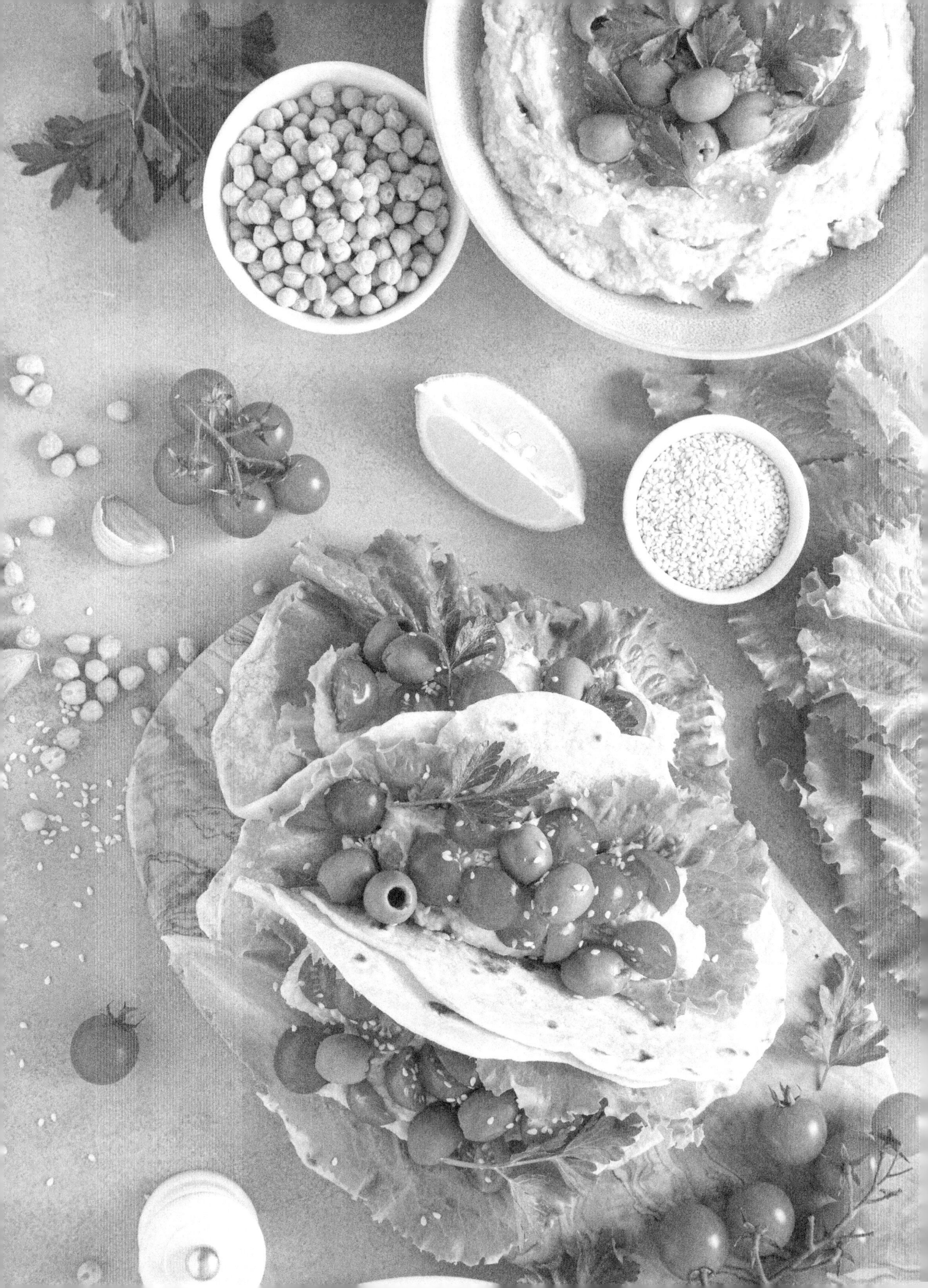

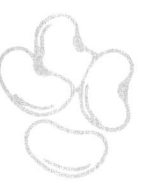

MEDITERRANEAN LETTUCE CHICKPEA WRAPS

NUTRITIONAL VALUE

- Calories- 443 kcal
- Carbohydrates-49.3g
- Proteins-16.9g
- Fats-25g

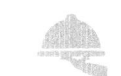

SERVINGS - 6

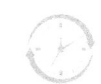

TIME - 28 min

INGREDIENTS

- ¼ cup tahini
- ¼ cup olive oil
- 1 tsp lemon zest
- ¼ cup lemon juice
- 1 ½ tsp maple syrup
- ¾ kosher salt
- ½ tsp paprika
- 2 cups boiled chickpeas
- ½ cup roasted peppers
- ½ cup thinly sliced shallots
- 12 large lettuce leaves
- ½ cup toasted chopped almonds
- 2 tbsp chopped parsley

INSTRUCTIONS

1. In a mixing bowl add lemon zest, oil, tahini, lemon juice, maple syrup, salt, and pepper. Mix all the ingredients.
2. To the same mixing bowl add chickpeas, peppers, and shallots.
3. Open lettuce leaves and place the chickpeas mixture into the center of lettuce leaves. Also, add some almonds and parsley in the center.
4. Wrap lettuce leaves in such a way that filling gets closed in the lettuce wraps.
5. Blanch the rolls for 5 minutes and serve.

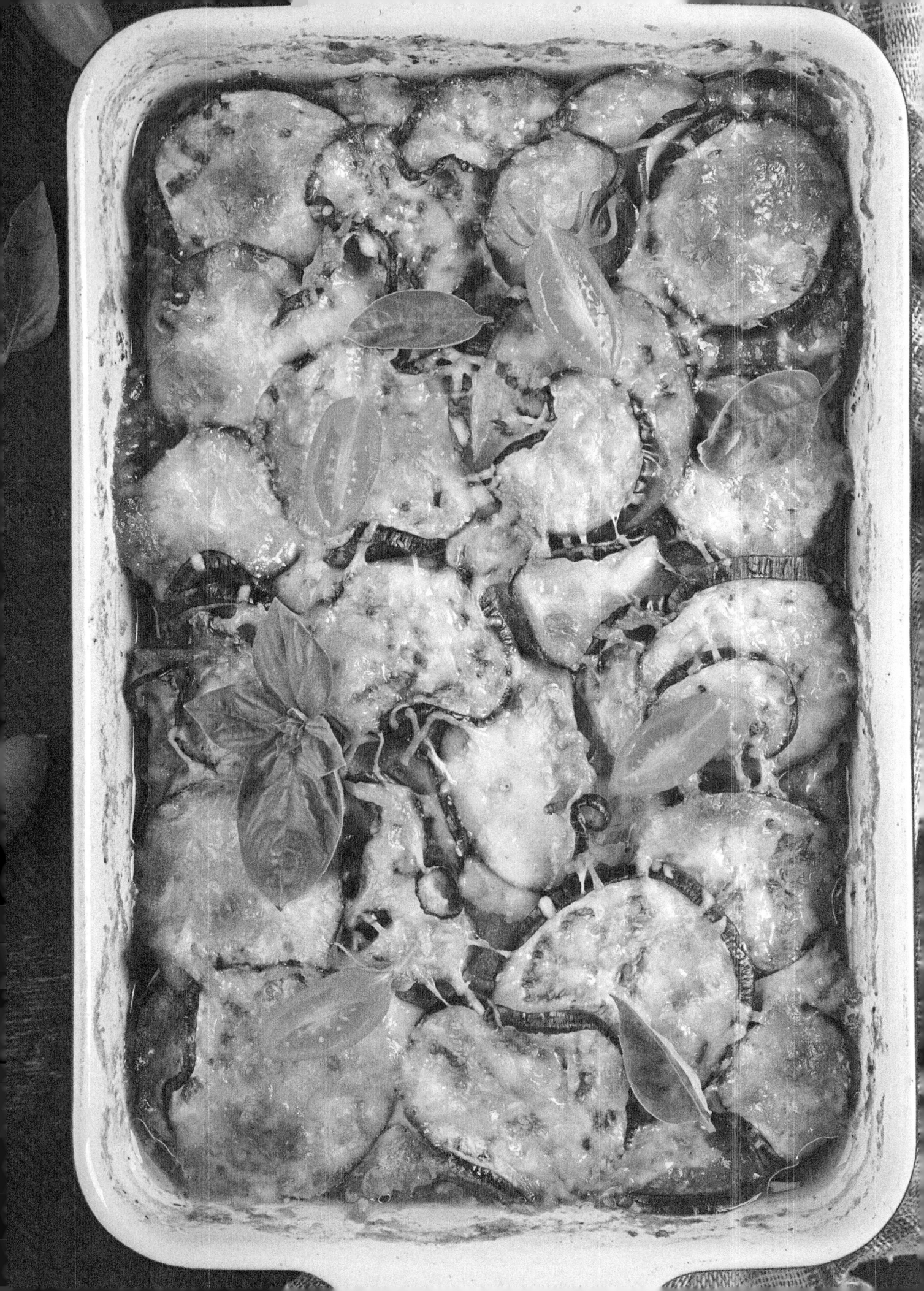

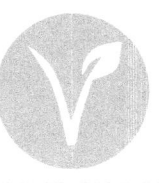

EGGPLANT LASAGNA

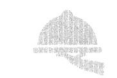

SERVINGS - 4

TIME - 1 Hrs

NUTRITIONAL VALUE

- Calories- 712 kcal
- Carbohydrates- 9.2g
- Proteins-42.8g
- Fats-53.8g

INGREDIENTS

- 2 diced eggplants
- 2 tbsp butter
- ½ diced onion
- 1/3 cup marinara sauce
- 1 cup ricotta cheese
- 2 tbsp chopped parsley
- 2 tbsp chopped mint
- ½ cup ground beef
- Salt as per taste
- Black pepper as per taste
- 1 large egg
- ¾ cup mozzarella cheese
- 2/3 cup parmesan cheese

INSTRUCTIONS

1. Take the eggplant and slice them into uniform slices. Brush these slices with oil and display them onto a baking dish. Bake the eggplant slices for 10 minutes at at 400 degree Fahrenheit (200 degrees Celsius).
2. Cool the eggplant slices and set them aside.
3. Now take a skillet and add some butter to it. Sauté onions into the melted butter and add ground beef into it. Cook the beef for few minutes until it changes its color.
4. Now add the marinara sauce in it and again cook it until it's tender and soft. And some salt and pepper as per your taste.
5. In another mixing bowl add ricotta cheese, salt, pepper, chopped herbs, and an egg. Mix everything to make a creamy sauce.
6. Take a heat-resistant glass baking dish and spread a layer of marinara sauce at the top followed by a layer of 1/3rd eggplant slices on top of it.
7. Spread a layer of ricotta cheese on top of the eggplant slices followed by a layer of beef filling.
8. Again place the layer of eggplant slices and repeat this process until three layers are formed.
9. Finally spread a good amount of mozzarella cheese and parmesan cheese and bake the lasagna for 30 minutes at 356 degree Fahrenheit (180 degrees Celsius).

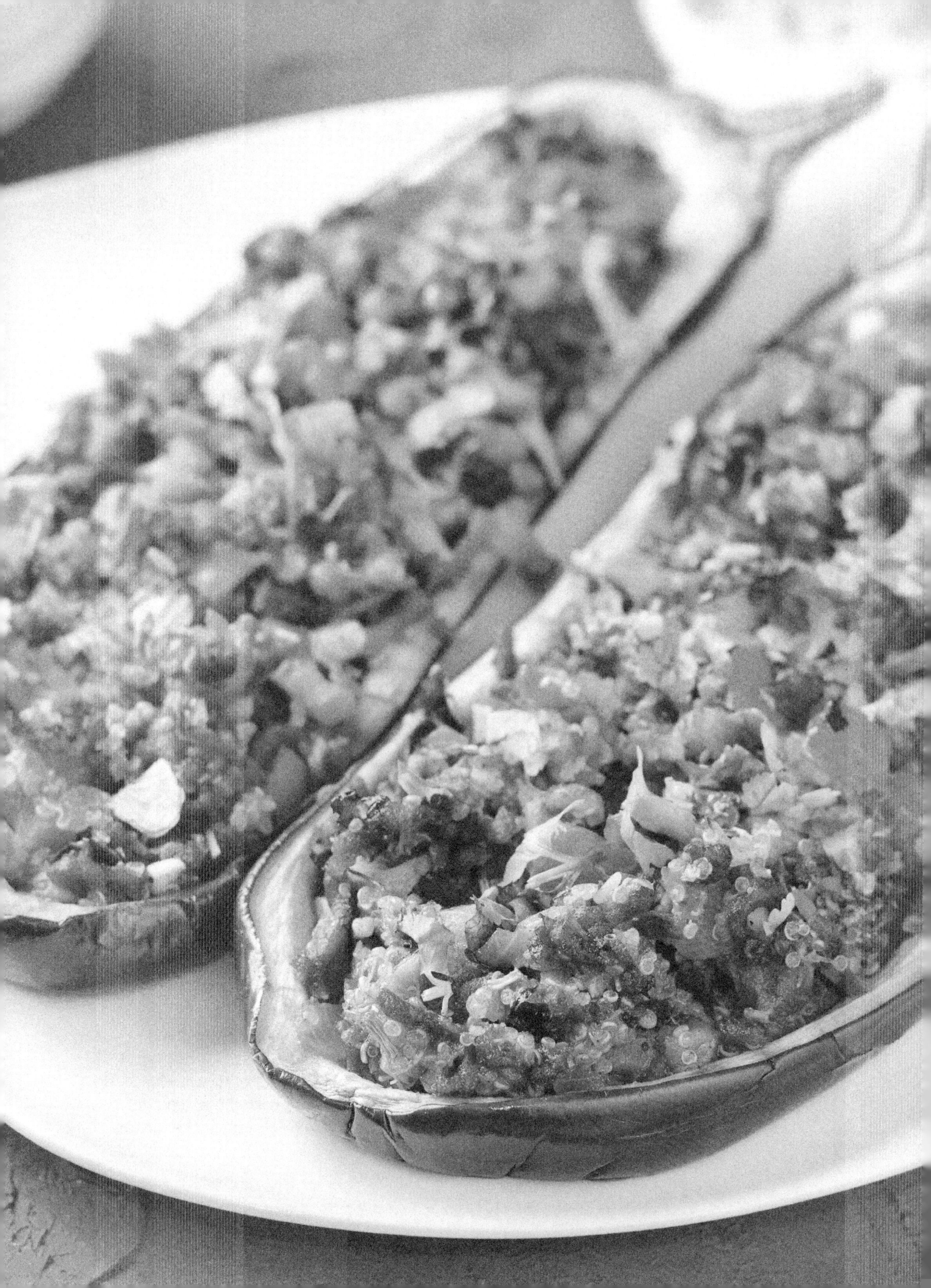

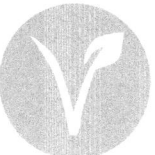

QUINOA STUFFED EGGPLANT WITH TAHINI SAUCE

SERVINGS - 2

TIME - 30 min

NUTRITIONAL VALUE

- Calories- 342 kcal
- Carbohydrates-18.1g
- Proteins-13.8g
- Fats-64g

INGREDIENTS

- 1 eggplant
- 2tbsp olive oil
- 1 diced red onion
- 1 cup chopped mushrooms
- 6 chopped tomatoes
- 1 tbsp tomato puree
- 2 minced garlic cloves
- ½ cup cooked quinoa
- 1 tbsp tahini sauce
- 1 tsp lemon juice
- ½ tsp garlic powder
- ½ tsp ground cumin
- 1 tbsp chopped parsley
- Water as required

INSTRUCTIONS

1. Cut eggplant into half and scoop out a bit of eggplant from the center to make a cavity inside. Toss eggplant pieces in olive oil with some salt and pepper.
2. Bake eggplants for 20 minutes at at 425 degrees Fahrenheit (220 degree Celsius).
3. In a large skillet add olive oil and sauté onion and mushrooms into it for 5 minutes. Now add tomatoes, tomato puree, cumin, salt, pepper, cooked quinoa, and some water. Cook all the ingredients together.
4. Stuff this quinoa mixture into the cavity of eggplant and again bake it for 20 minutes at 375 degrees Fahrenheit.
5. To make the sauce, combine tahini with some water, lemon juice, garlic powder, and salt.
6. Drizzle tahini sauce over the stuffed eggplant and serve.

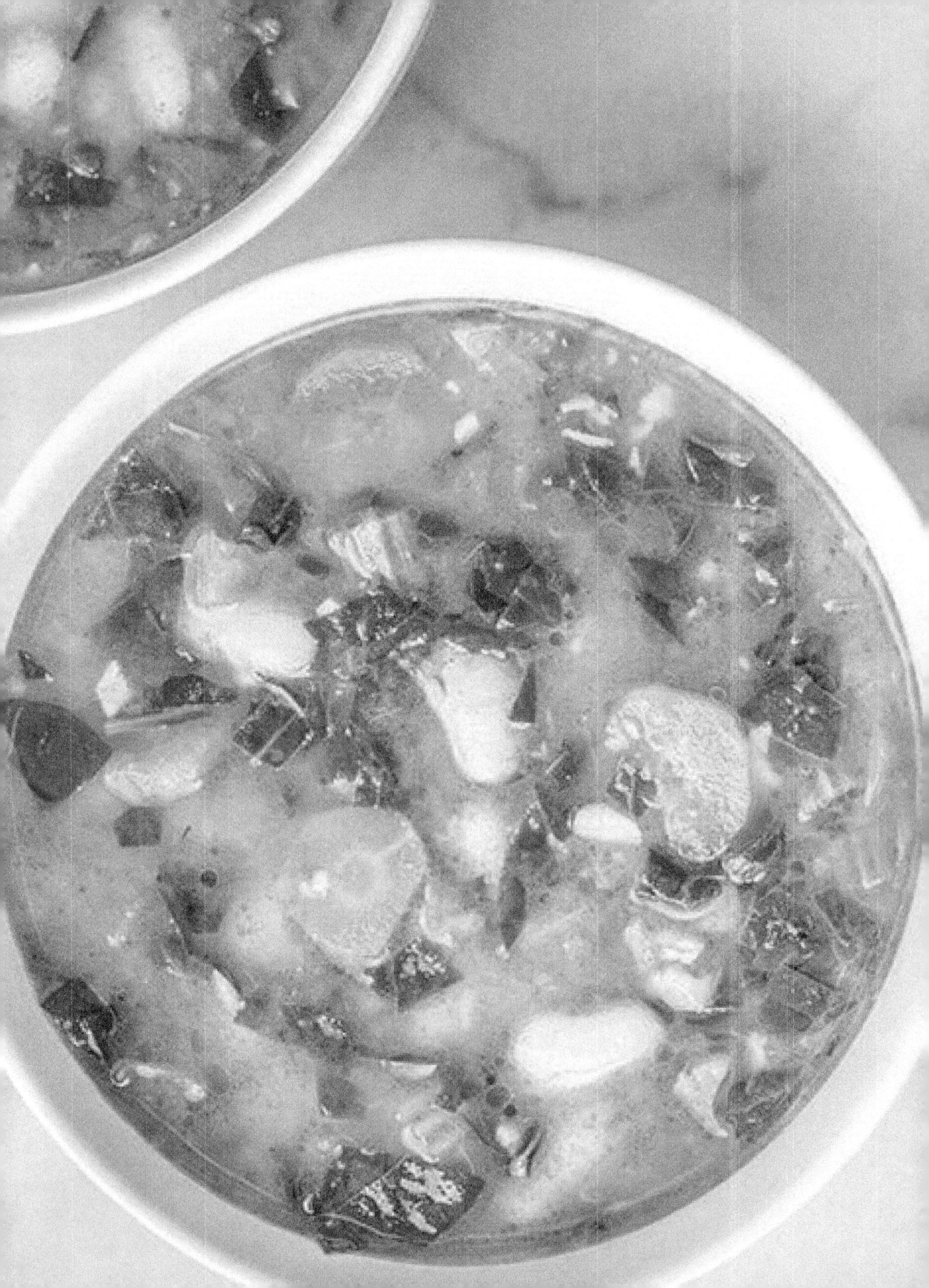

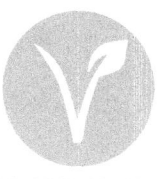

FLAT BELLY SOUP

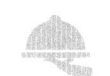

SERVINGS - 6

TIME - 20 min

 NUTRITIONAL VALUE

- Calories-161 kcal
- Carbohydrates-28.6g
- Proteins-5g
- Fats-4.6g

 INGREDIENTS

- 1 tbsp olive oil
- 2 cups chopped butternut squash
- 1 cup chopped onion
- ¾ cup sliced parsnips
- 3 tsp chopped garlic
- 1 tsp chopped ginger
- 1 tsp ground turmeric
- ½ tsp ground cumin
- ½ tsp salt
- 6 cups low sodium vegetable broth
- 1 cup stewed tomatoes
- 3 cups chopped rainbow chard
- 1 cup chickpeas
- 1 tbsp apple cider vinegar
- 1 tbsp chopped parsley

 INSTRUCTIONS

1. In a deep pot add oil along with squash, onions, and parsnips. Cook these things for 15 minutes.
2. To the pot add tomatoes and broth and bring it to boil.
3. Simmer the contents for 10 minutes until all the vegetables are tender.
4. Also, add chard and chickpeas and stir the mixture for 2 minutes.
5. Add some vinegar and sprinkle some chopped parsley onto the top of the serving bowl.

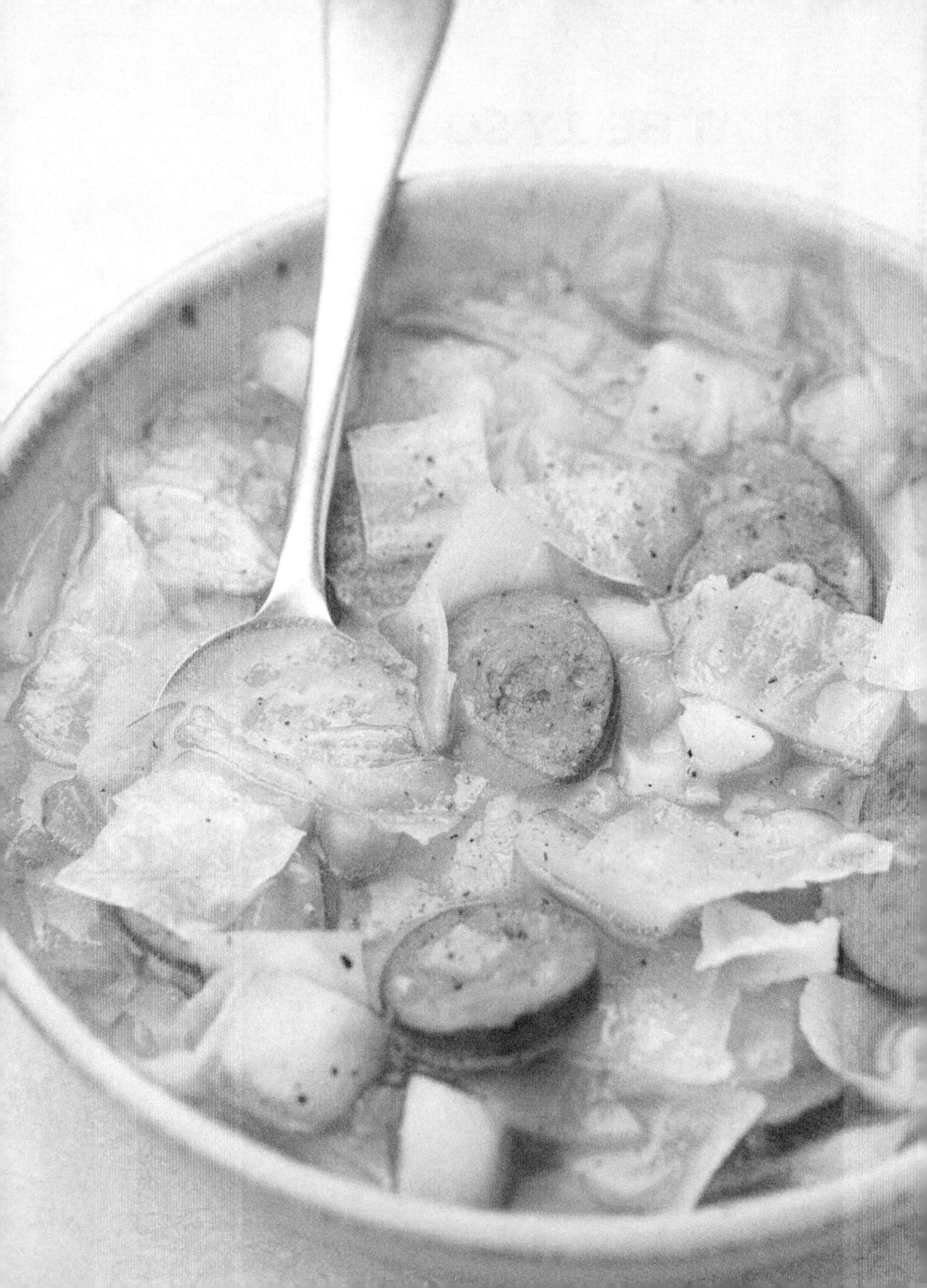

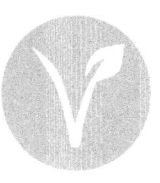

CABBAGE SOUP

SERVINGS - 8

TIME - 25 min

 NUTRITIONAL VALUE

- Calories-57 cal
- Carbohydrates-13g
- Proteins-2g
- Fats-2g

 INGREDIENTS

- 8 cup vegetable broth
- 1 chopped onion
- 3 minced garlic cloves
- 4 cups cabbage chunks
- 3 sliced carrots
- 3 sliced celery stalks
- ½ tsp kosher salt
- ½ tsp black pepper
- ½ tsp oregano
- ½ tsp dried basil
- 1 cup diced tomatoes

 INSTRUCTIONS

1. Add vegetable broth, tomatoes, onions, garlic, cabbage, carrots, celery, salt, pepper, oregano, basil, and stir the mixture well.
2. Boil the ingredients and simmer for 20 minutes. Serve hot!

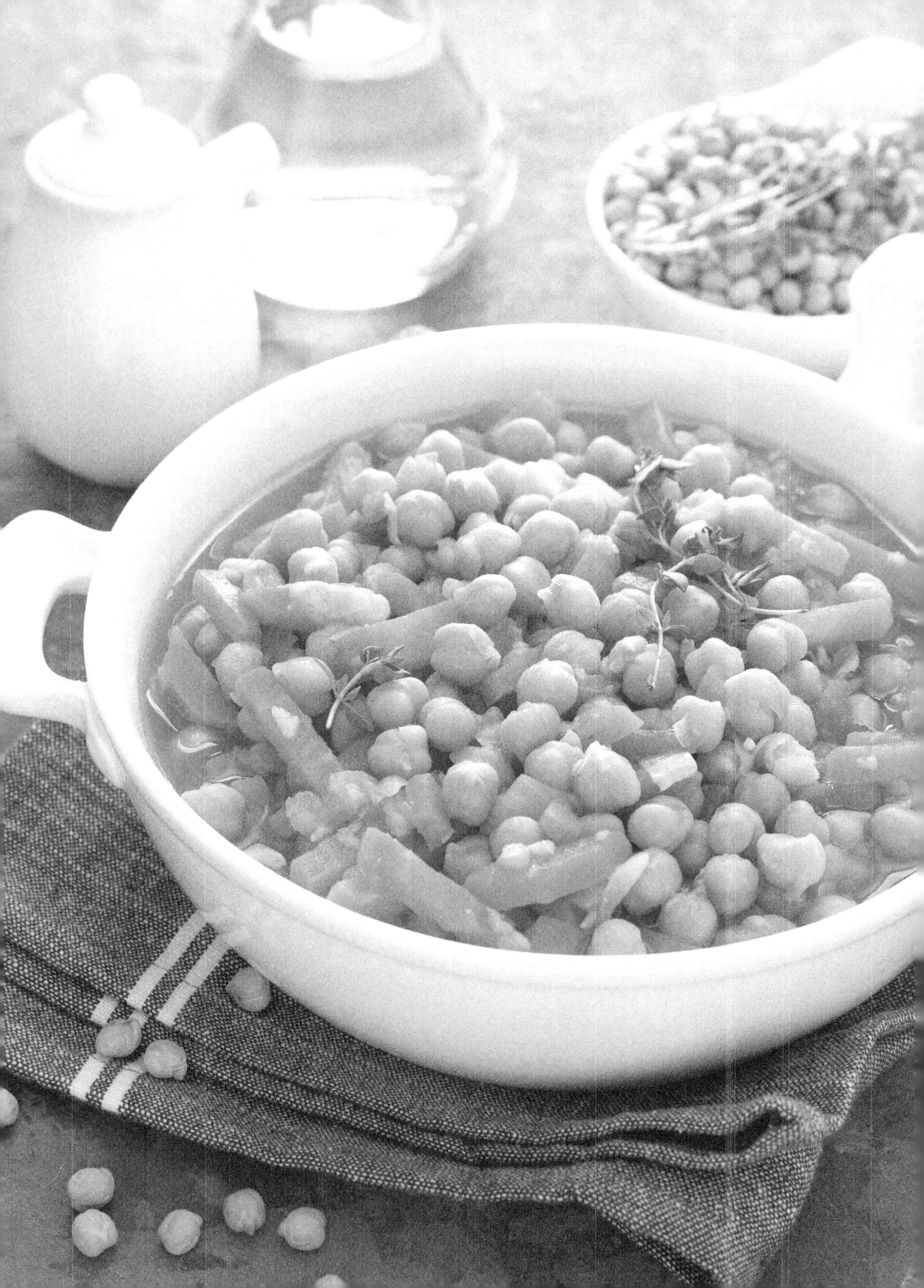

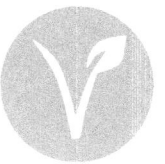

CHICKPEA TOMATO AND SPINACH CURRY

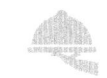

SERVINGS - 6

TIME - 30 min

 NUTRITIONAL VALUE

- Calories-204 kcal
- Carbohydrates-20g
- Proteins-11g
- Fats-7g

 INGREDIENTS

- 1 chopped onion
- 2 chopped garlic cloves
- 1 tbsp grated ginger
- 6 ripe tomatoes
- ½ tsp oil
- 1 tsp ground cumin
- 2 tsp ground coriander
- 1 tsp turmeric
- 1 pinch chili flakes
- 1 tsp yeast
- 4 tbs red lentils
- 6 tbsp coconut cream
- 1 broccoli head
- 2 cups chickpeas
- ½ cup baby spinach
- 1 tbsp lemon juice
- 1 tbsp toasted sesame seeds
- 1 tbsp chopped cashews

 INSTRUCTIONS

1. Blitz onion, garlic, ginger, and tomatoes into a smooth paste with the help of a food processor.
2. Heat oil in a deep pot and add in some spices. Add paste and yeast into it.
3. Cook everything for 2 min and add lentils along with some coconut milk.
4. Break broccoli into small florets and add them to the pot.
5. Also add some chickpeas, spinach, lemon juice, and drizzle some sesame seeds and cashew on top.
6. Serve with cauliflower rice.

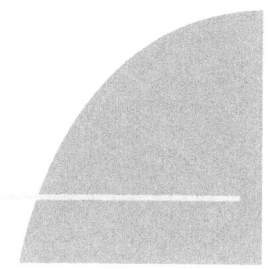

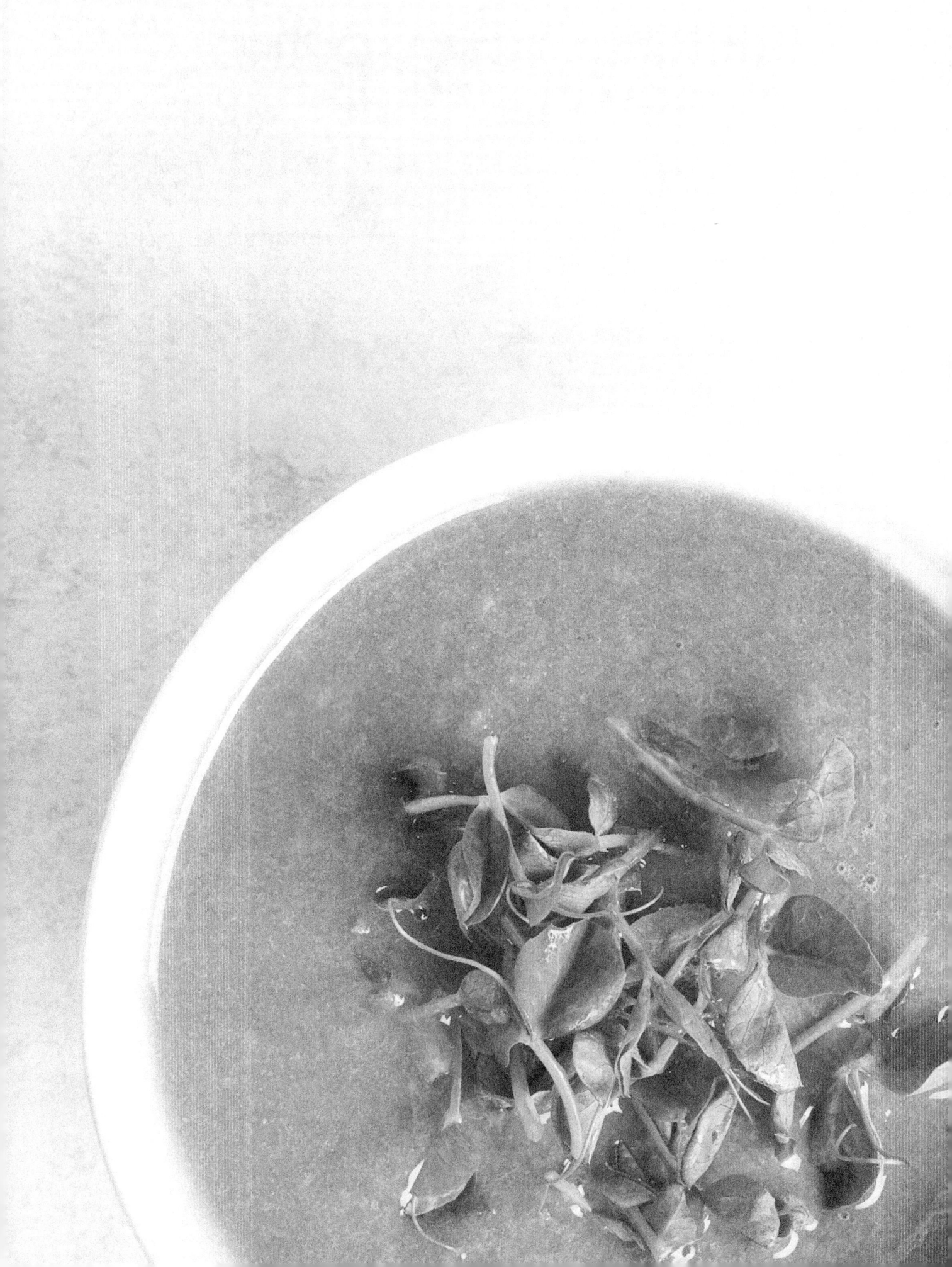

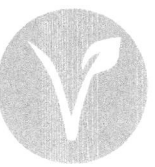

BROCCOLI AND KALE GREEN SOUP

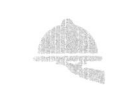

SERVINGS - 2

TIME - 20 min

 NUTRITIONAL VALUE

- Calories-182 kcal
- Carbohydrates-14g
- Proteins-10g
- Fats-8g

 INGREDIENTS

- 2 cups vegetable stock
- 1 tbsp olive oil
- 2 sliced garlic
- 1 tbsp sliced ginger
- ½ tsp ground coriander
- ½ tsp ground turmeric
- 1 pinch salt
- ¾ cup of courgettes
- ½ cup broccoli
- ½ cup kale
- 2 tbsp chopped parsley

 INSTRUCTIONS

1. In a deep pan add oil, garlic, ginger, coriander, and turmeric, salt, and fry them for 2 minutes. Add a splash of water.
2. Add courgettes to the spice mixture and cook them for 3 minutes. Now add vegetable stock and simmer the contents for 15 minutes.
3. Add kale, broccoli, lime juice and again cook for 5 minutes.

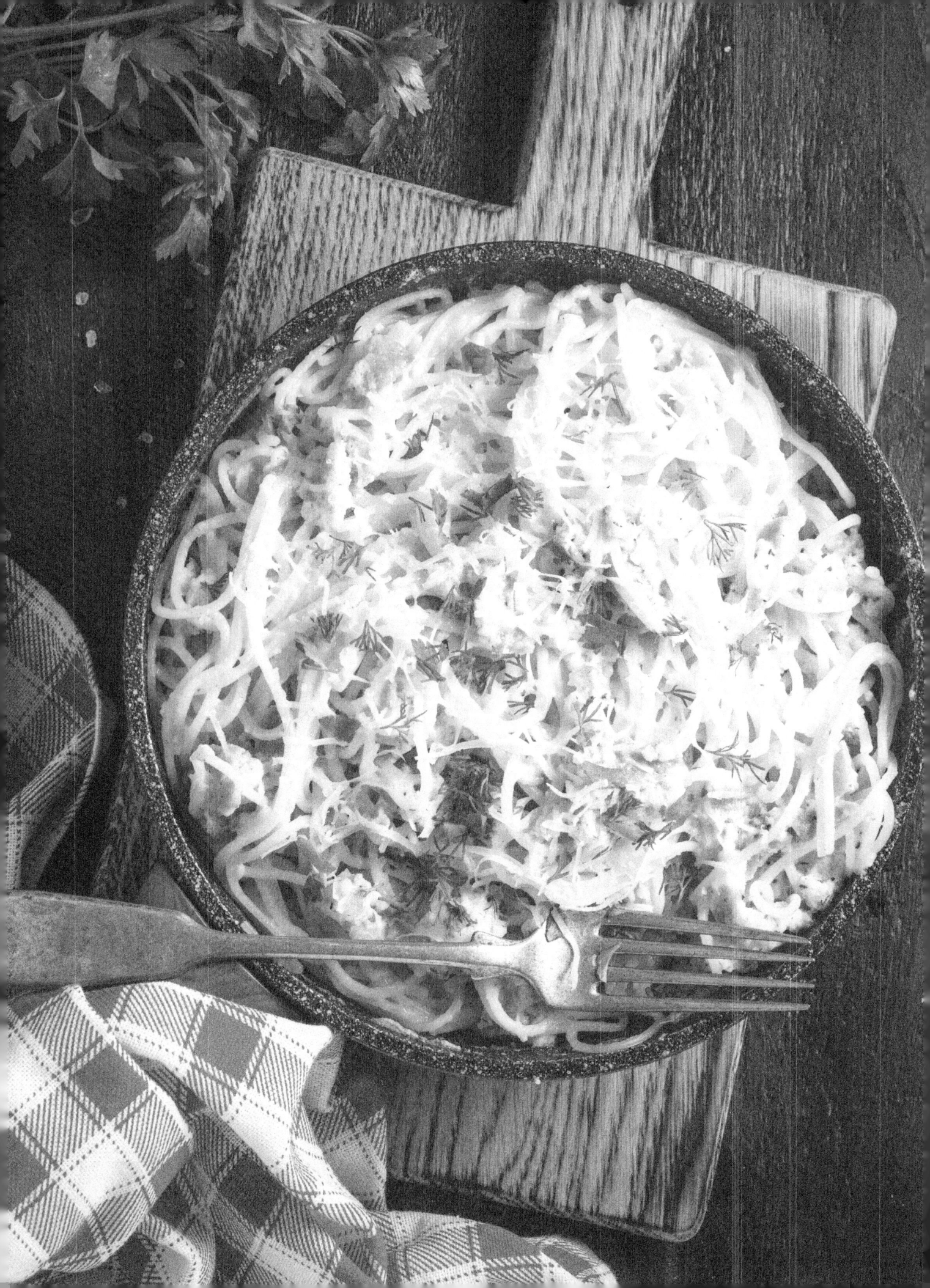

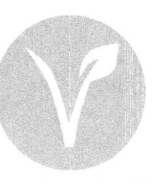

PEA SPINACH CARBONARA

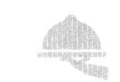

SERVINGS - 3

TIME - 20 mins

 NUTRITIONAL VALUE

- Calories-506 cal
- Carbohydrates-40g
- Proteins-36.7g
- Fats-38g

 INGREDIENTS

- 2 tbsp olive oil
- ½ cup bread crumbs
- 1 small minced garlic
- 8 tbsp grated parmesan cheese
- 3 tbsp chopped parsley
- 3 large egg yolks
- ½ tsp ground pepper
- ¼ tsp salt
- 1 cup fresh linguine
- 8 cups baby spinach
- 1 cup peas

 INSTRUCTIONS

1. In pan roast breadcrumbs along with garlic. Add the contents into a separate bowl and 2 tbsp of parmesan cheese in it. Set it aside.
2. Mix remaining parmesan cheese with egg yolks, salt, and pepper in another separate bowl.
3. In a separate pan, cook paste long with some peas and spinach. Drain all the things and reserve the drained water.
4. Transfer the cooked pasta mixture into the pan and add egg yolk mixture with reserved drained water and cook it for 3 minutes.
5. Finally, top the dish with roasted breadcrumbs and enjoy.

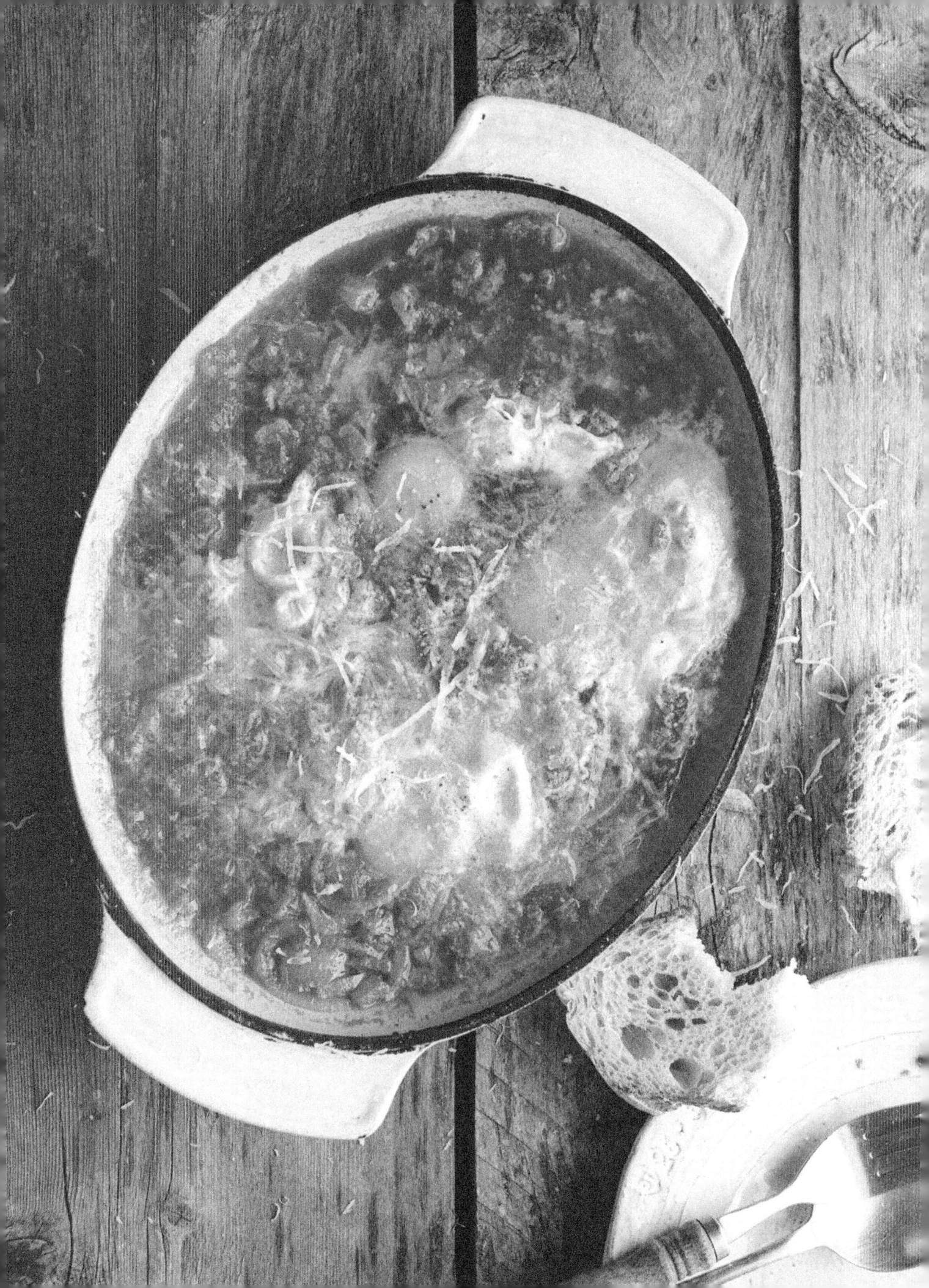

ACQUACOTTA

SERVINGS - 5

TIME - 40 mins

NUTRITIONAL VALUE

- Calories-239 kcal
- Carbohydrates-17g
- Proteins-14g
- Fats-12g

INGREDIENTS

- 3 tbsp olive oil
- 3 chopped celery stalks
- 2 small chopped carrots
- 1 chopped red onion
- 2 chopped garlic cloves
- 2 tsp thyme leaves
- ¼ cup mushrooms
- 1 cup plum tomatoes
- 3 cups vegetable stock
- 6 eggs

INSTRUCTIONS

1. Heat some oil in a large pot and fry carrots, celery, onions, garlic, mushrooms, and thyme for a few minutes.
2. Add some tomatoes and cook them for the next 10 minutes. Also, add some stock. Cook the mixture for 20 minutes.
3. Prepare poached eggs by breaking eggs one by one in boiling water.
4. Prepare your serving bowl by adding some soup and placing a poached egg on top of it.

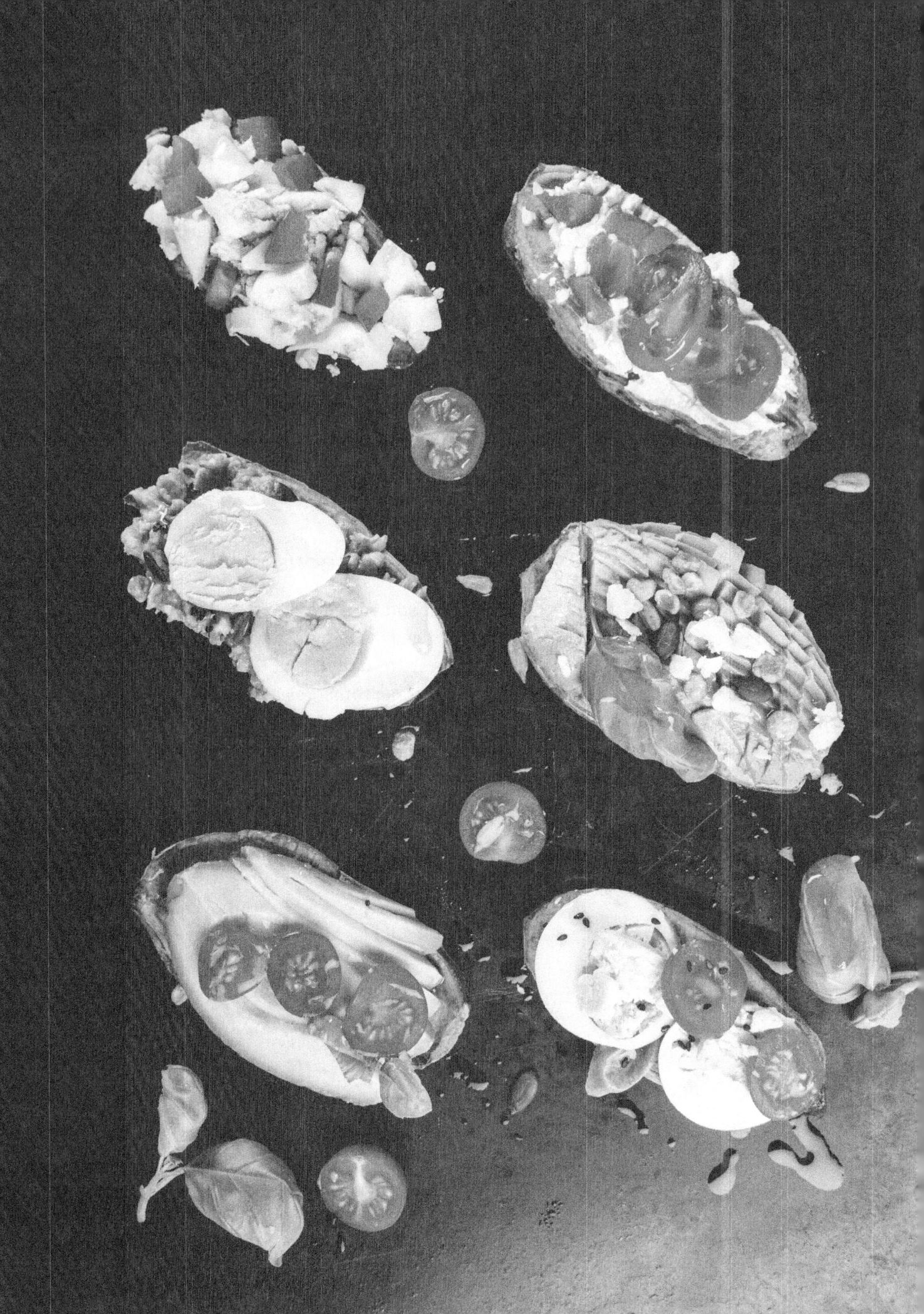

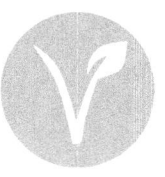

SWEET POTATO TOAST

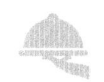

SERVINGS - 5

TIME - 40 mins

 NUTRITIONAL VALUE

- Calories-22 kcal
- Carbohydrates-5g
- Proteins-1g
- Fats-1g

 INGREDIENTS

- 1 sweet potato
- Olive oil

 INSTRUCTIONS

1. Cut sweet potato into 1 inch thick slices.
2. Brush oil on both sides.
3. Place slices on the baking sheet and bake them for 30 minutes.

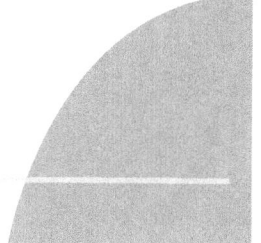

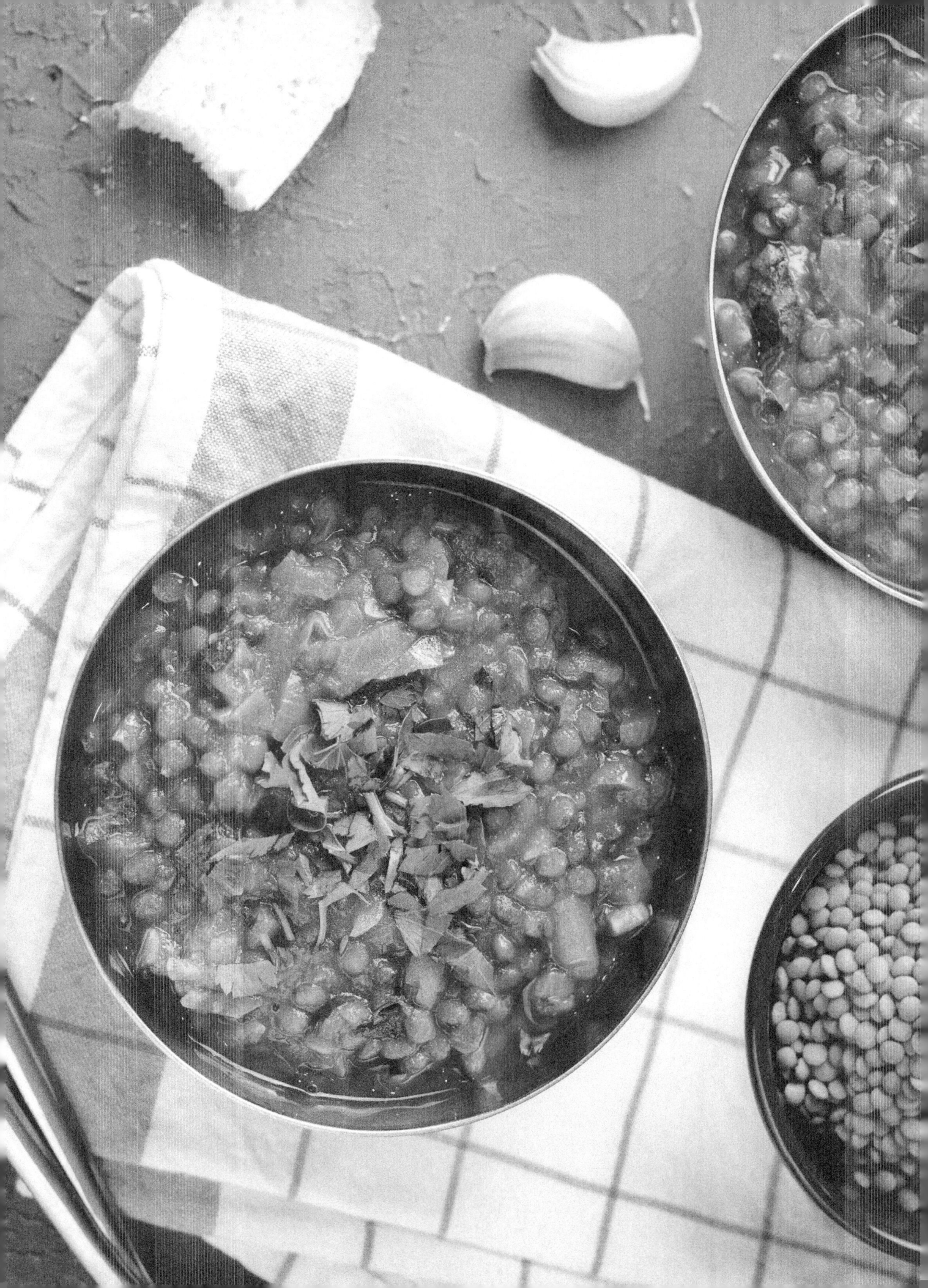

SLOW COOKER MEDITERRANEAN STEW

SERVINGS - 2

TIME - 6hr 40 mins

 NUTRITIONAL VALUE

- Calories- 452 kcal
- Carbohydrates-43.9g
- Proteins-15.7g
- Fats-14.7g

 INGREDIENTS

- 2 cups roasted diced tomatoes
- 3 cups vegetable broth
- 1 cup chopped onions
- ¾ cup chopped carrots
- 4 minced garlic clove
- 1 tsp oregano
- ¾ tsp salt
- ½ tsp crushed pepper
- ¼ tsp ground pepper
- 1 cup chickpeas
- 1 bunch chopped and steamed kale
- 1 tbsp lemon juice
- 3 tbsp olive oil
- 2 tbsp basil leaves
- 6 lemon juice

 INSTRUCTIONS

1. Take a slow cooker and add tomatoes, vegetable broth, salt, red pepper, black pepper, oregano, onion, carrot. Cook all these ingredients in a slow cooker for at least 6 hours.
2. Measure ¼ cup of cooking liquid and add 2 tbsp chickpeas into it. Smash chickpeas into the liquid.
3. Add smashed chickpeas liquid, kale, lemon juice, whole chickpeas, and salt into the slow cooker. Cover the slow cooker and cook for another 30 minutes.
4. Garnish your stew with basil and lemon wedges and serve it hot.

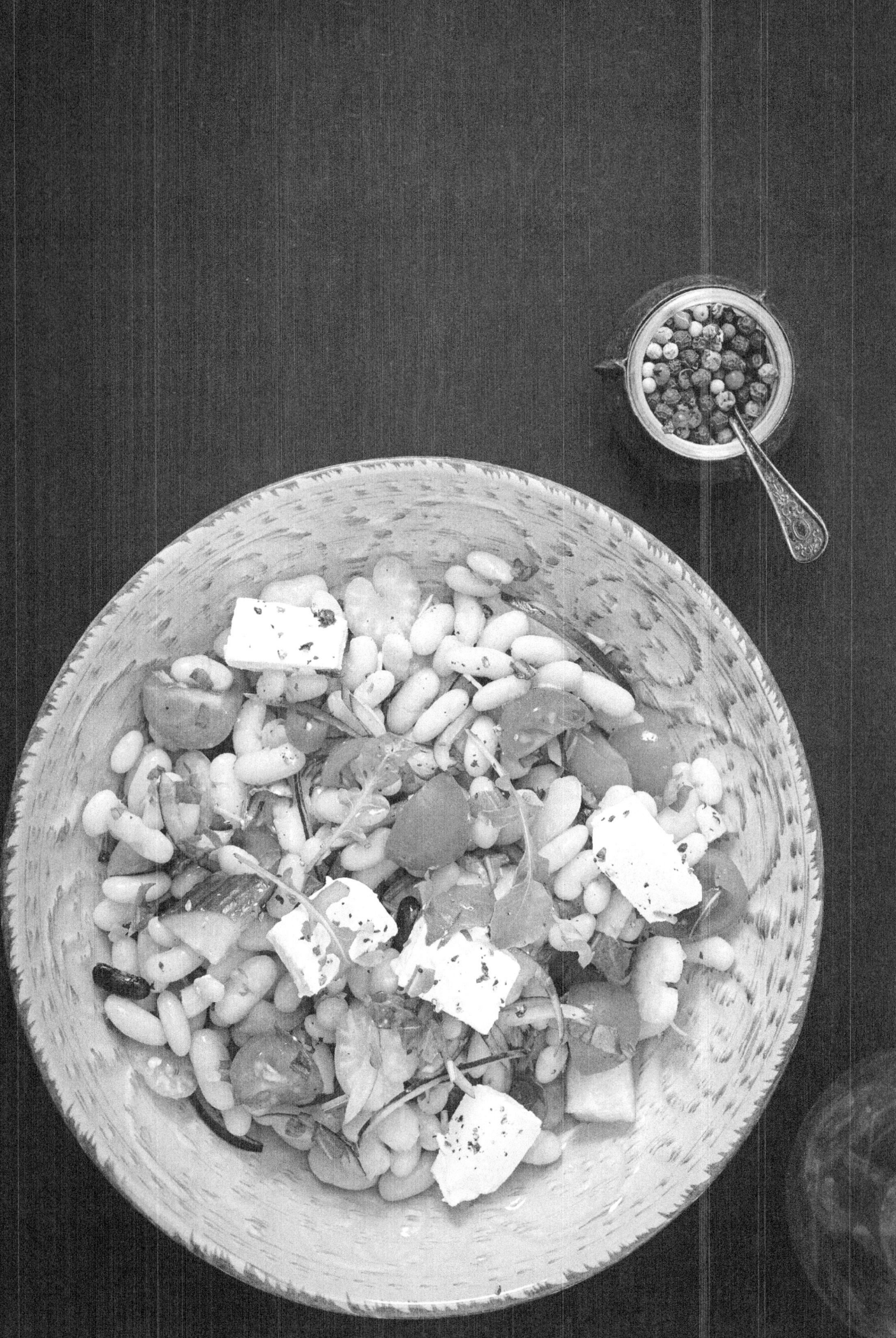

TOMATO CUCUMBER WHITE BEAN SALAD

SERVINGS - 4

TIME - 10 mins

 NUTRITIONAL VALUE

- Calories-345kcal
- Carbohydrates-37.2g
- Proteins-12.9g
- Fats-13.6g

 INGREDIENTS

- ½ cup basil leaves
- ¼ cup olive oil
- 3 tbsp vinegar
- 1 tbsp chopped shallots
- 2 tsp mustard
- 1 tsp honey
- ¼ tsp salt
- ¼ tsp ground black pepper
- 1 cups mixed greens
- 1 cup boiled cannellini beans
- 1 cup halved cherry tomatoes
- 1 cup diced cucumbers

 INSTRUCTIONS

1. In a food processor add basil leaves, olive oil, vinegar, mustard, honey, salt, and black pepper to make a paste.
2. In a mixing bowl add shallots, cucumber, mixed greens, cannellini beans, and cherry tomatoes.
3. Drizzle over some sauce to prepare the salad.

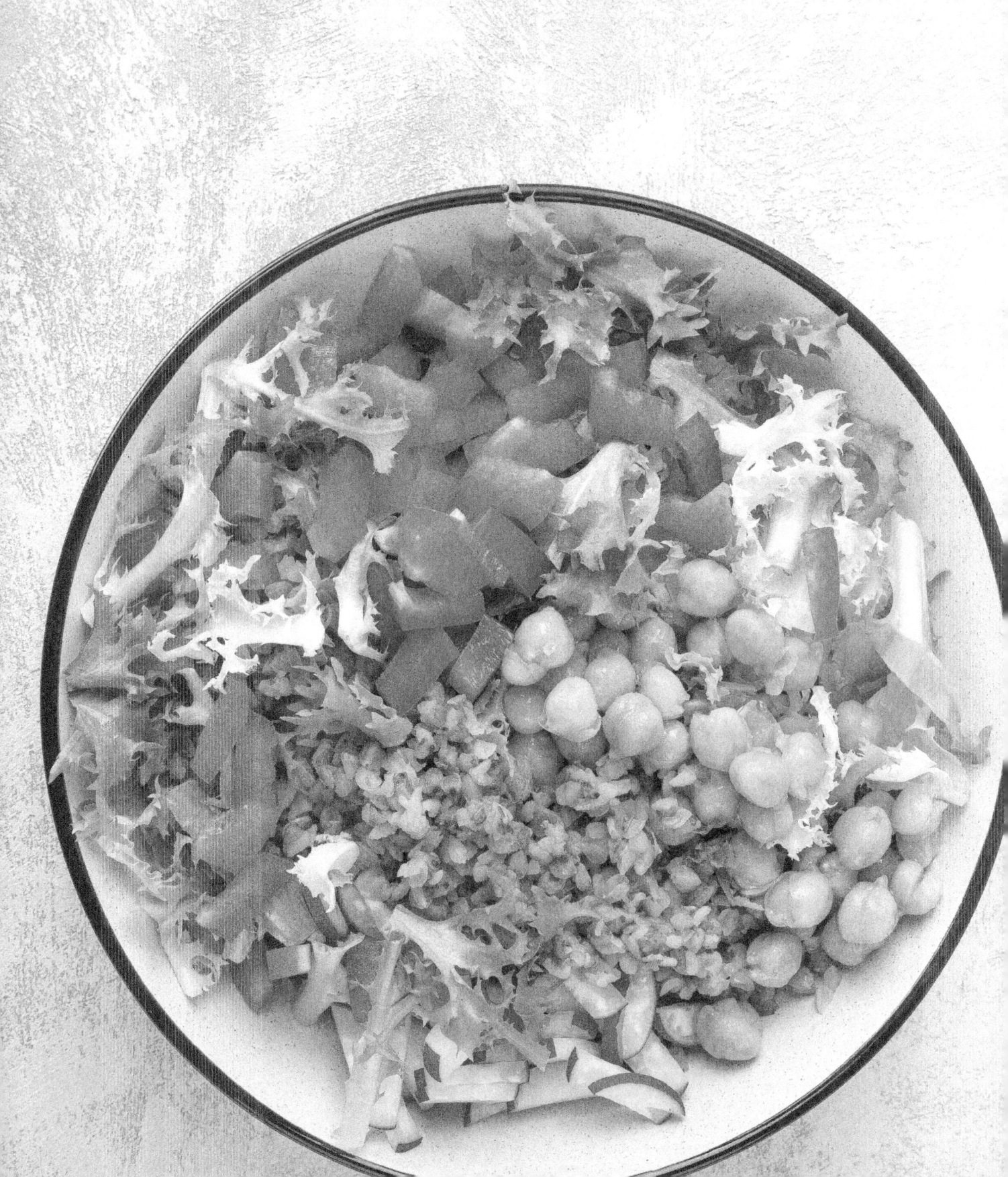

COUSCOUS AND CHICKPEA SALAD

SERVINGS - 1

TIME - 5 mins

NUTRITIONAL VALUE

- Calories-1019 cal
- Carbohydrates-188.9g
- Proteins-44.3g
- Fats-18.9g

INGREDIENTS

- 1 cup chopped kale
- ¾ cup couscous
- 2/3 cup boiled chickpeas
- 4 tbsp vinegar

INSTRUCTIONS

1. In a mixing bowl add kale along with some couscous, chickpeas, and vinegar.
2. Toss everything together and prepare the quick and healthy salad.

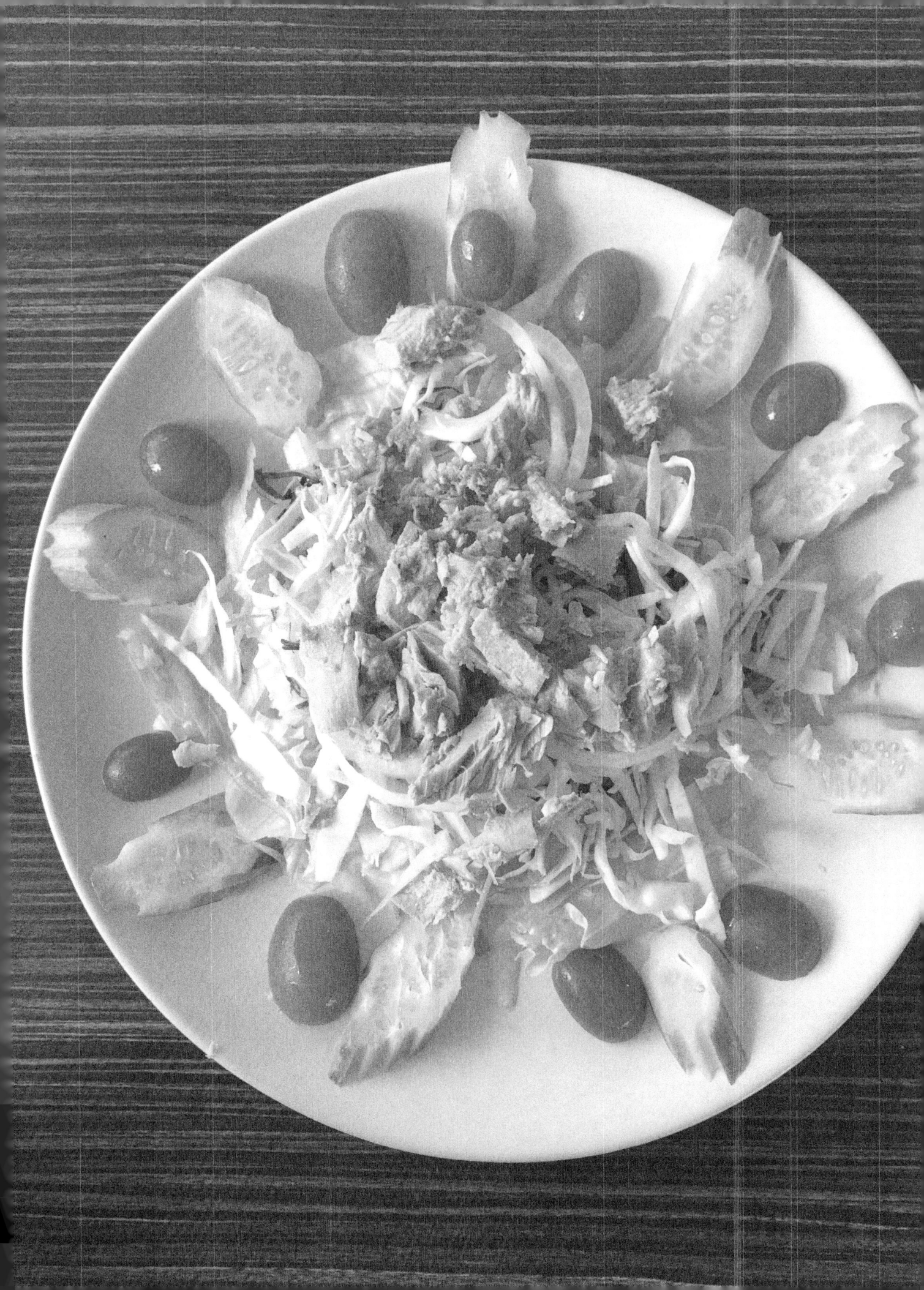

MEDITERRANEAN TUNA SPINACH SALAD

SERVINGS - 2

TIME - 10 mins

NUTRITIONAL VALUE

- Calories-276 cal
- Carbohydrates-15.7g
- Proteins-5.2g
- Fats-9.3g

INGREDIENTS

- 1 ½ tbsp. tahini
- 1 ½ tbsp lemon juice
- 1 ½ tbsp water
- 2 cups cooked tuna pieces
- 4 olives cut into slices
- 2 tbsp crumbled feta cheese
- 2 tbsp chopped parsley
- 2 cups baby spinach
- 1 diced orange

INSTRUCTIONS

1. Add lemon juice, tahini, and water in a whisking bowl and mix to form a dressing.
2. In another bowl add tuna pieces, loves, feta cheese, parsley, spinach, and some diced orange pieces.
3. Drizzle some dressing onto the salad and enjoy!

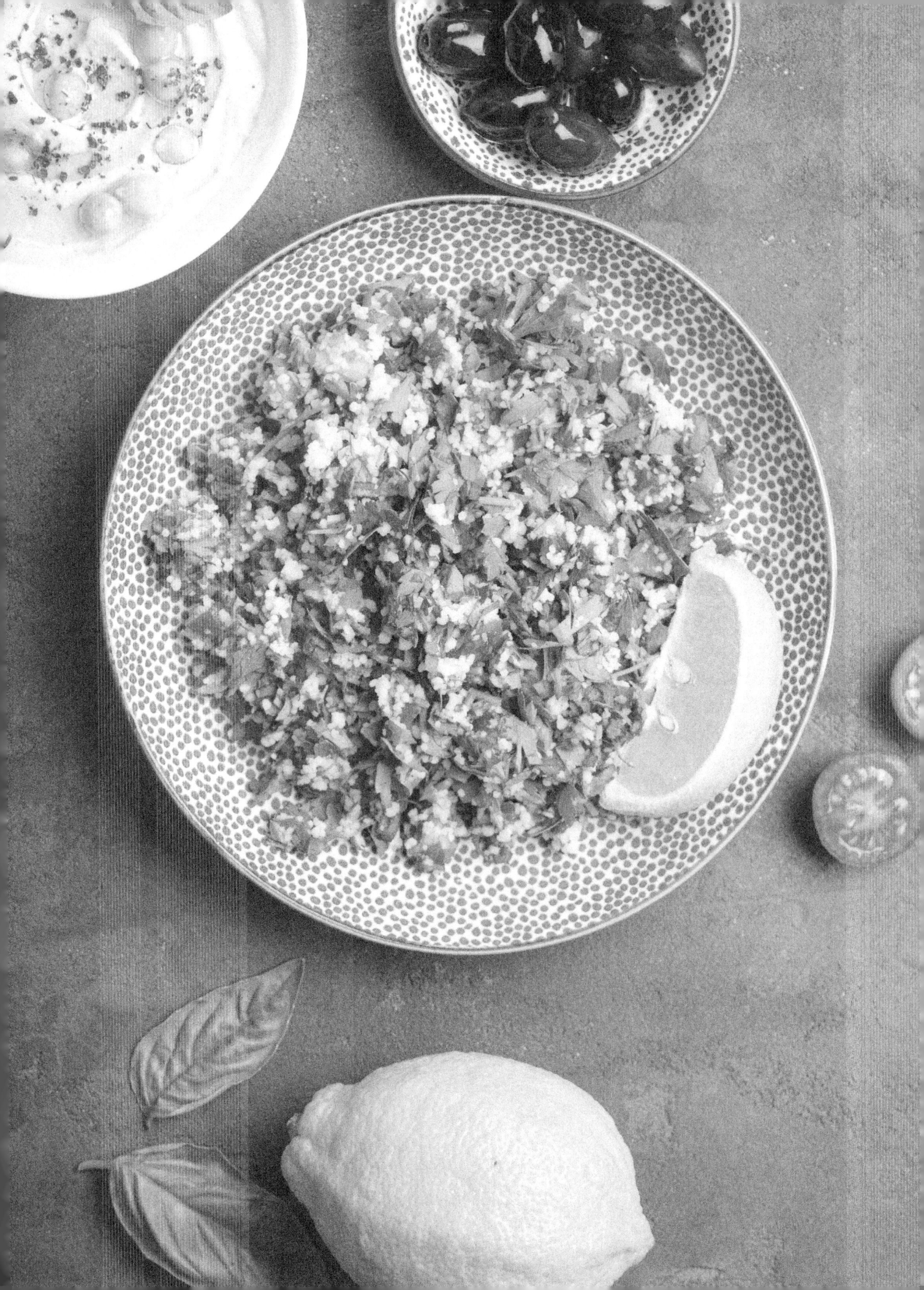

 # TABBOULEH SALAD

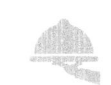
SERVINGS - 3

TIME - 5 mins

 NUTRITIONAL VALUE

- Calories- 123 kcal
- Carbohydrates-11g
- Proteins-3.2g
- Fats-5.6g

 INGREDIENTS

- 3 cups chopped parsley
- 3 diced tomatoes
- 2 squeezed lemons
- 1 tsp salt
- ½ tsp black pepper
- 1 small diced onion
- ½ tsp fresh mint
- 1 tbsp olive oil

 INSTRUCTIONS

1. In a large mixing bowl add parsley, tomatoes, mint, and onions.
2. Toss the ingredients with some lemon juice, salt, and pepper.
3. Finally, drizzle over some olive oil, and enjoy!

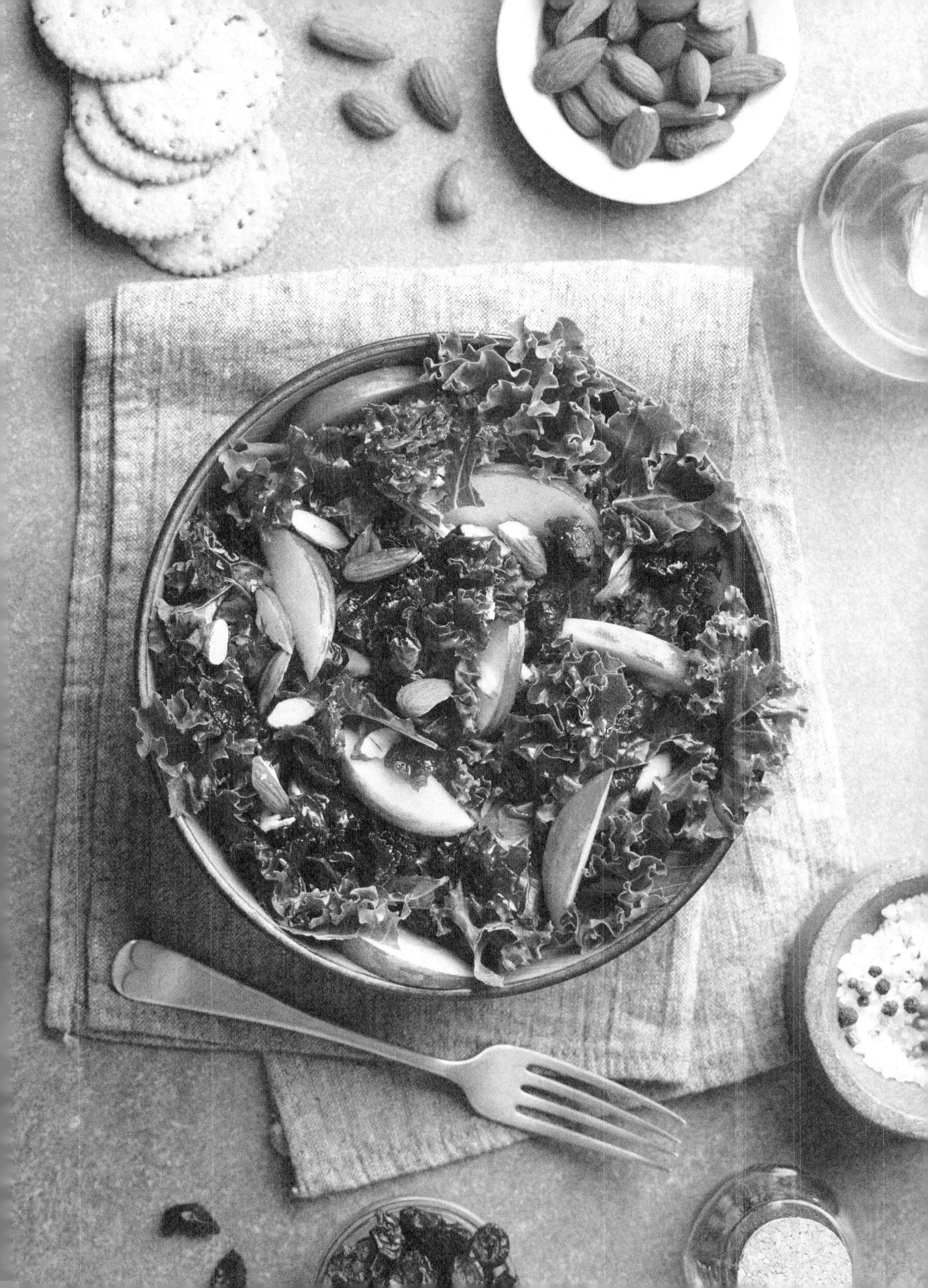

FRESH KALE SALAD WITH TAHINI DRESSING

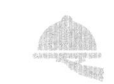

SERVINGS - 3 **TIME - 15 mins**

 NUTRITIONAL VALUE

- Calories-294 kcal
- Carbohydrates-34g
- Proteins- 48g
- Fats- 38g

 INGREDIENTS

- 4-6 cups Kale
- 2 tbsp lemon juice
- 12 pieces of vegan falafel
- Tahini for dressing
- ½ red onion
- 1 cup white beans
- 1 jalapeno
- 2 pita bread slices

 INSTRUCTIONS

1. Bake vegan falafel pieces in the oven until they are nice golden crispy.
2. Roughly cut kale leaves into pieces.
3. In a large mixing bowl add kale along with some lemon juice and nicely toss the leaves into the citrus environment.
4. Add white beans, sliced red onion, chopped jalapenos, and pita bread pieces into the same mixing bowl and mix the contents nicely.
5. Now add crispy falafel balls along with some tahini dressing to elevate this salad for lunch.

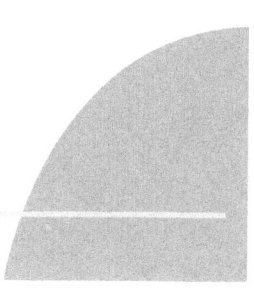

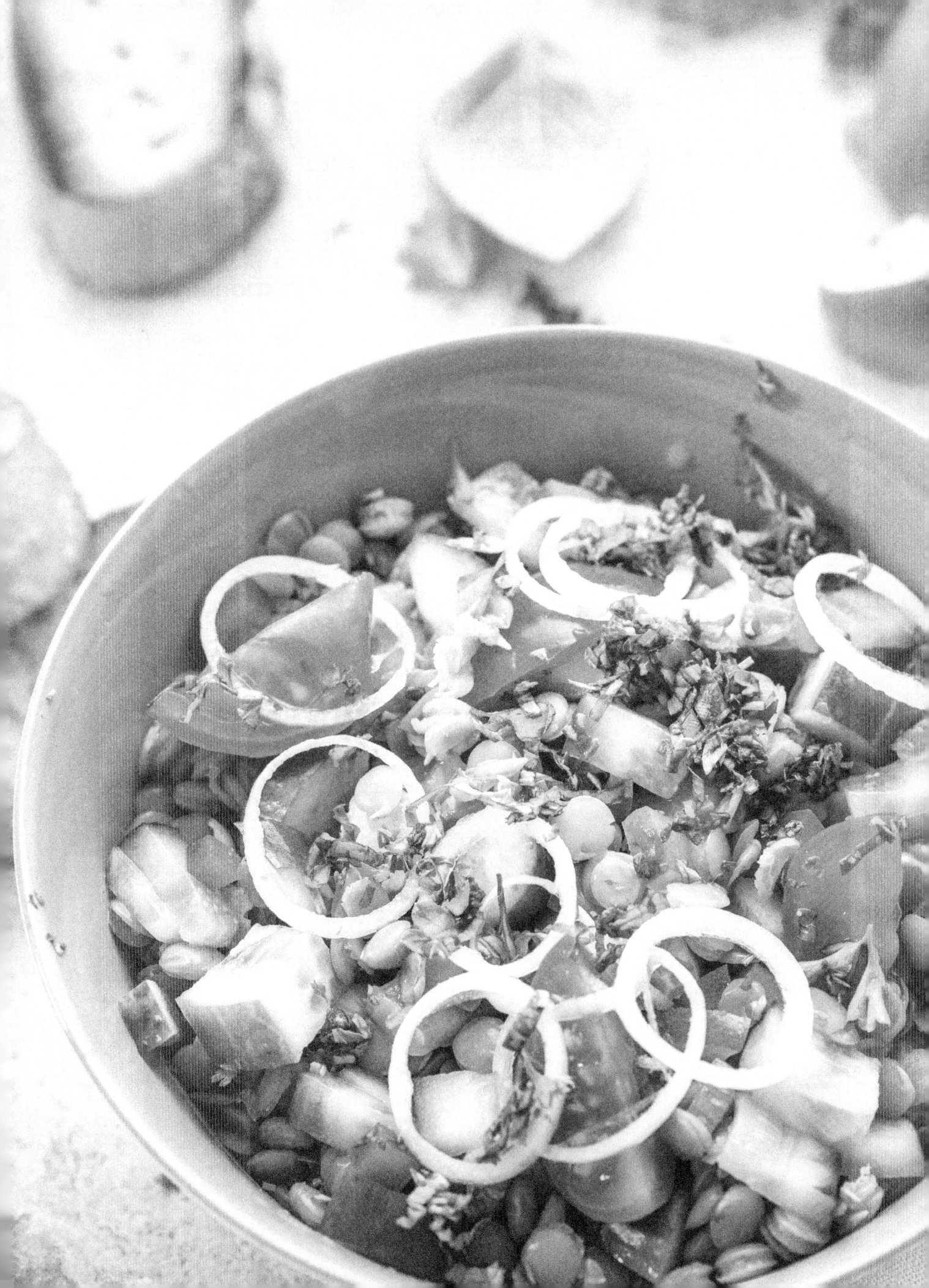

LENTIL SALAD

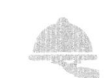

SERVINGS - 2

TIME - 30 mins

 NUTRITIONAL VALUE

- Calories-221 kcal
- Carbohydrates- 33g
- Proteins-14g
- Fats-7g

 INGREDIENTS

- 1 cup French lentils
- 1 bay leaf
- ¼ cup chopped red onion
- 3 quartered radishes
- 2 chopped celery stalks
- ½ chopped red bell pepper
- ¼ cup chopped parsley
- 1 tbsp Crumbled feta cheese
- 3 tbsp lemon juice
- 1 tbsp olive oil
- 1 minced garlic clove
- Salt to taste

 INSTRUCTIONS

1. Prepare the dressing by combining salt, olive oil, lemon juice, and minced garlic clove. Set this dressing aside.
2. To prepare salad, first boil the lentils. For this purpose add lentils and bay leaf to a boiling pot of water and boil them for 15- 20 minutes.
3. Once the lentils are done add them to the bowl. To this bowl add chopped onions, celery, red bell pepper, radishes, parsley along with some feta cheese.
4. Combine all the ingredients well after drizzling dressing on top of the salad.

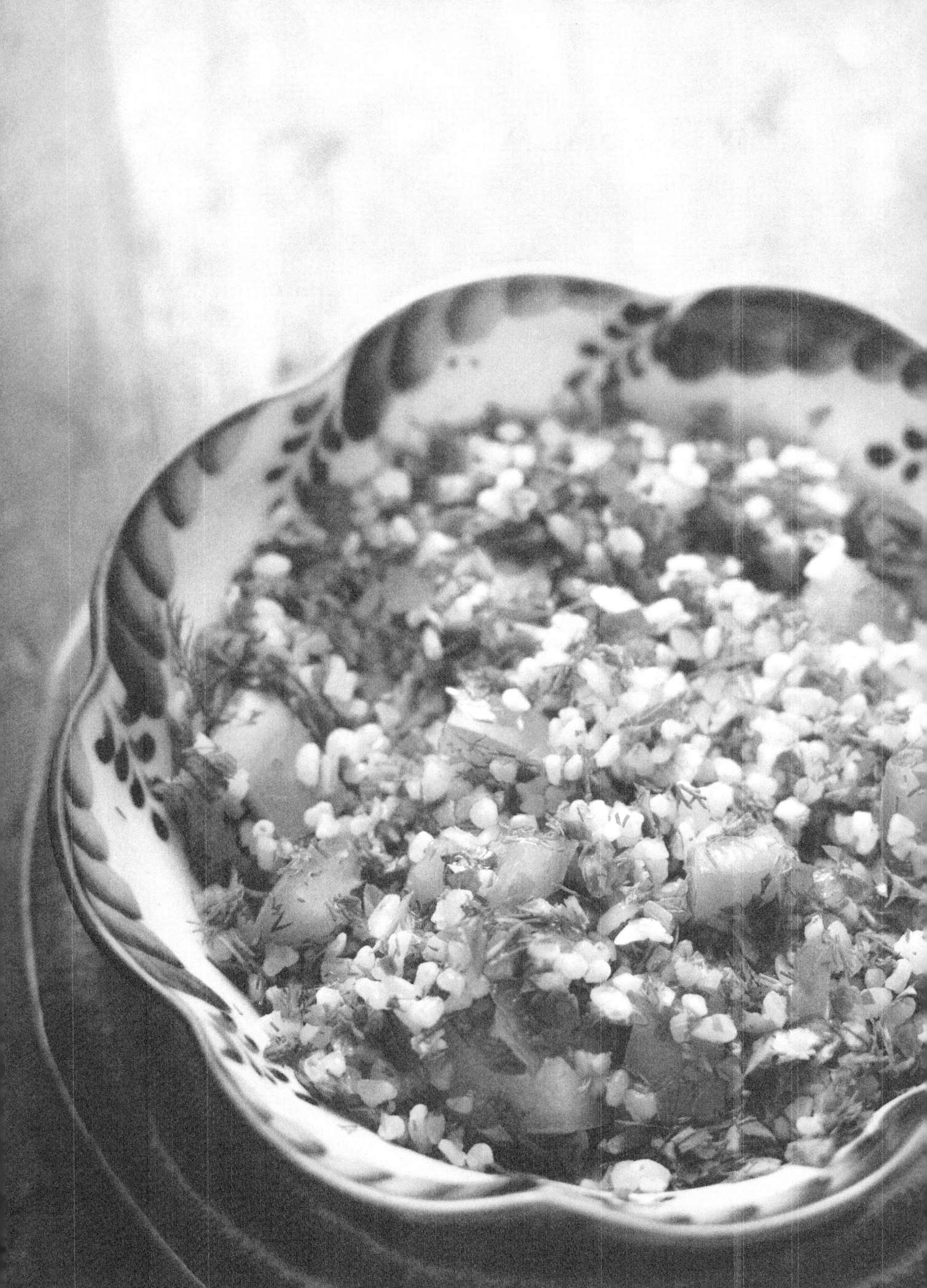

BULGUR SALAD WITH MARINATED FETA

SERVINGS - 2

TIME - 24 hrs

 NUTRITIONAL VALUE

- Calories-150 k cal
- Carbohydrates-15g
- Proteins-6g
- Fats-13g

 INGREDIENTS

- ½ cup feta cubes
- 1 tbsp lemon zest
- 1 tbsp chopped oregano leaves
- ½ tsp garlic powder
- 1 tsp ground black powder
- 1 cup bulgur salad
- 1 ½ cup boiling water
- ¼ cup minced mint leaves
- ¼ cup chopped parsley leaves
- 1 diced cucumber
- ½ cup diced tomato
- 2 tbsp lemon juice
- Salt to taste

 INSTRUCTIONS

1. Add lemon zest and oregano along with some garlic powder and black pepper into feta cubes. Transfer feta cubes into a jar and fill it with olive oil. Refrigerate the jar for at least 24 hrs.
2. Blanch bulgur in boiling water and boil it until tender. Drain it and set it aside.
3. Add parsley, mint, cucumber, tomatoes, and lemon juice to the bulgur.
4. Top your bulgur salad with marinated feta cheese to enhance the taste.

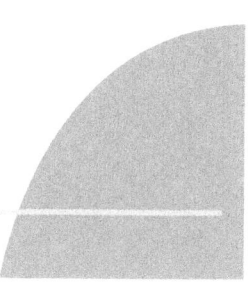

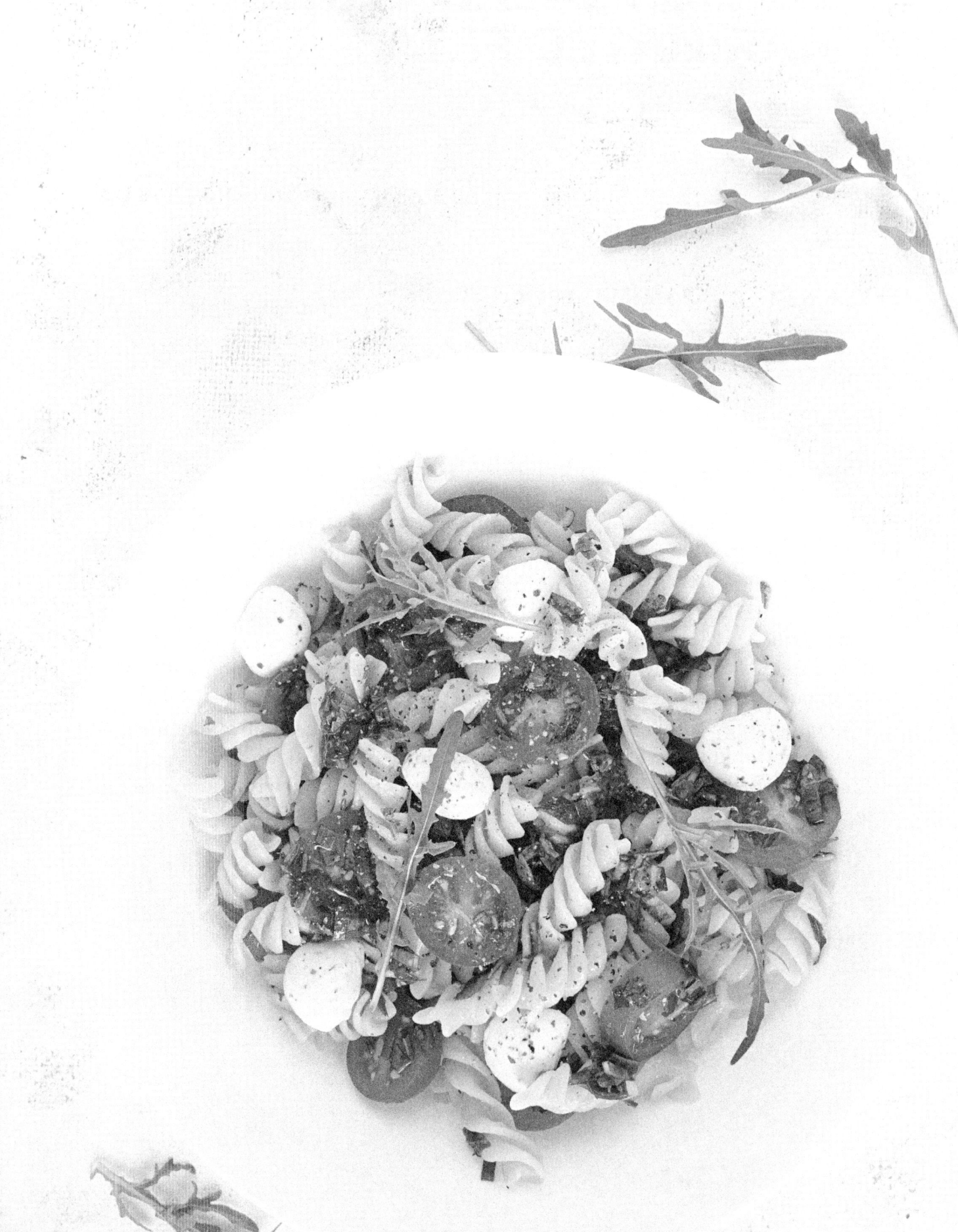

GLUTEN-FREE PASTA STYLE SALAD

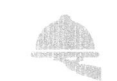

SERVINGS - 4

TIME - 50 mins

NUTRITIONAL VALUE

- Calories-465 kcal
- Carbohydrates-36g
- Proteins-7.5g
- Fats-40g

INGREDIENTS

- 1-pint cherry tomatoes
- 2 diced eggplants
- Avocado oil
- 1 tbsp chopped cilantro
- 1 tbsp chopped parsley
- 1 tbsp chopped dill
- 1 tbsp chopped mint
- 1 package brown rice spaghetti
- ¼ tsp granulated garlic + 4 large garlic cloves
- ¼ tsp red chili flakes
- ¼ tsp ground cumin
- 1 pinch black pepper
- 1 lemon zest
- ¼ cup lemon juice
- ¼ tsp salt
- ½ tsp mustard
- ¼ tsp granulated sugar
- ½ cup olive oil

INSTRUCTIONS

1. In a blender add garlic cloves, salt, lemon zest, lemon juice, mustard, sugar, and olive oil. Run blender at a very high speed to emulsify the mixture. Lemon dressing is ready!
2. To prepare pasta salad, take a large mixing bowl and mix cherry tomatoes, diced eggplants, salt, pepper, avocado oil, cumin, red chili flakes, and granulated garlic.
3. Empty the contents of the mixing bowl onto parchment paper-lined in a baking sheet and bake it for 35 minutes.
4. To combine salad with spaghetti, boil spaghetti by putting it in boiled water for 15 minutes.
5. Add spaghetti along with some baked veggies, lemon dressing, cilantro, parsley, dill, and mint.

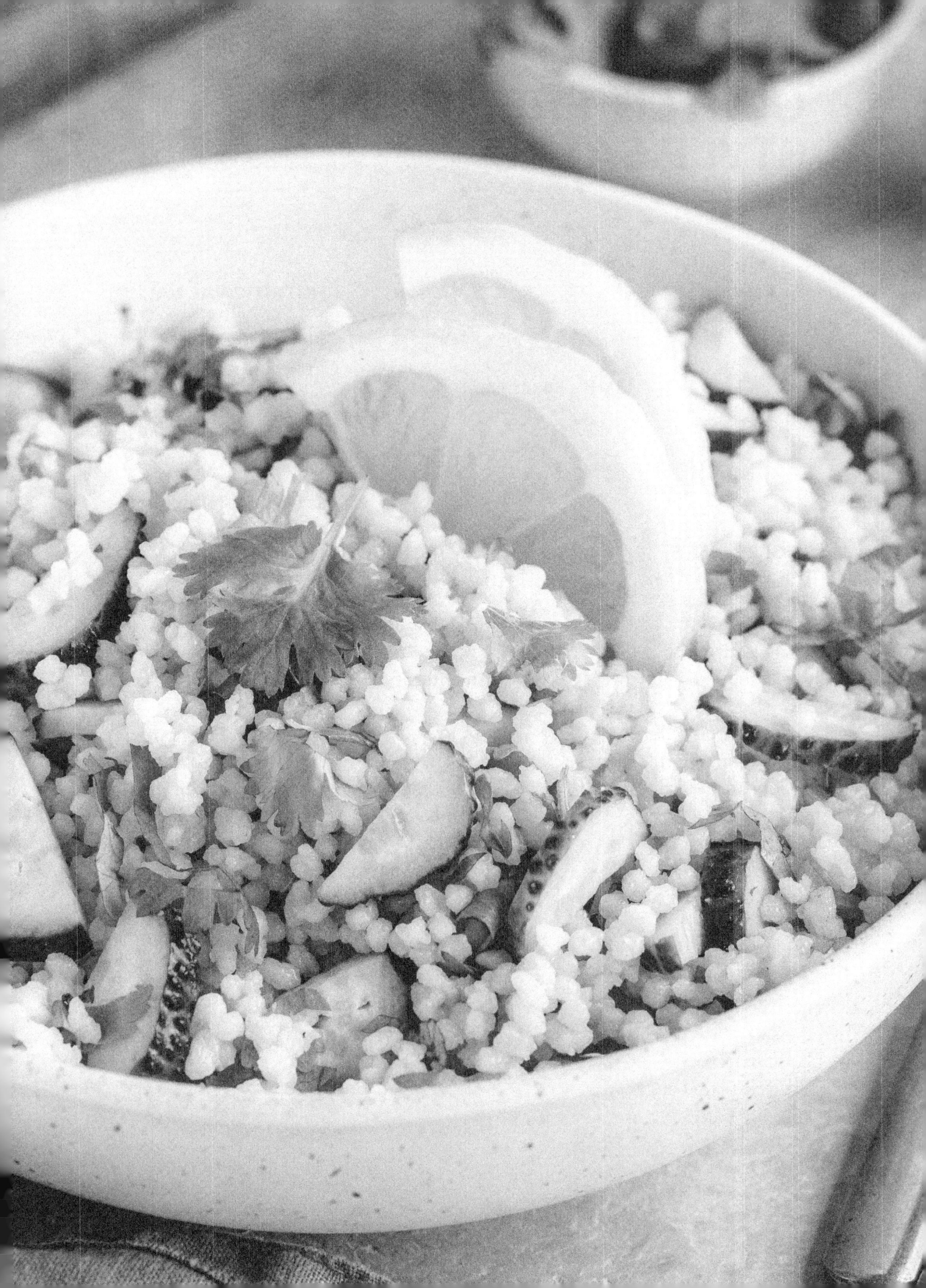

# LEMONY ORZO SALAD

SERVINGS - 2

TIME - 20 mins

 NUTRITIONAL VALUE

- Calories-598 kcal
- Carbohydrates-78g
- Proteins-23.4g
- Fats-42g

 INGREDIENTS

- 1 package orzo pasta
- 2 pints of baby spinach leaves
- 1 can garbanzo beans
- 1 diced cucumber
- ½ diced red onion
- 1 cup chopped basil leaves
- 1 cup chopped mint leaves
- 2 lemons
- ¼ cup olive oil
- Sea salt to taste
- Ground black pepper to taste
- ½ cup crumbled goat cheese

 INSTRUCTIONS

1. Boil pasta into boiling water and drain it after cooking.
2. In a mixing bowl add chopped spinach leaves, garbanzo beans, cucumber, red onion, chopped basil leaves, mint leaves, lemon zest, lemon juice, olive oil, salt, pepper, and some goat cheese. To the same bowl add orzo pasta and toss it gently into the mixing bowl. Herb's orzo is ready!

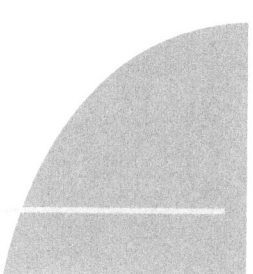

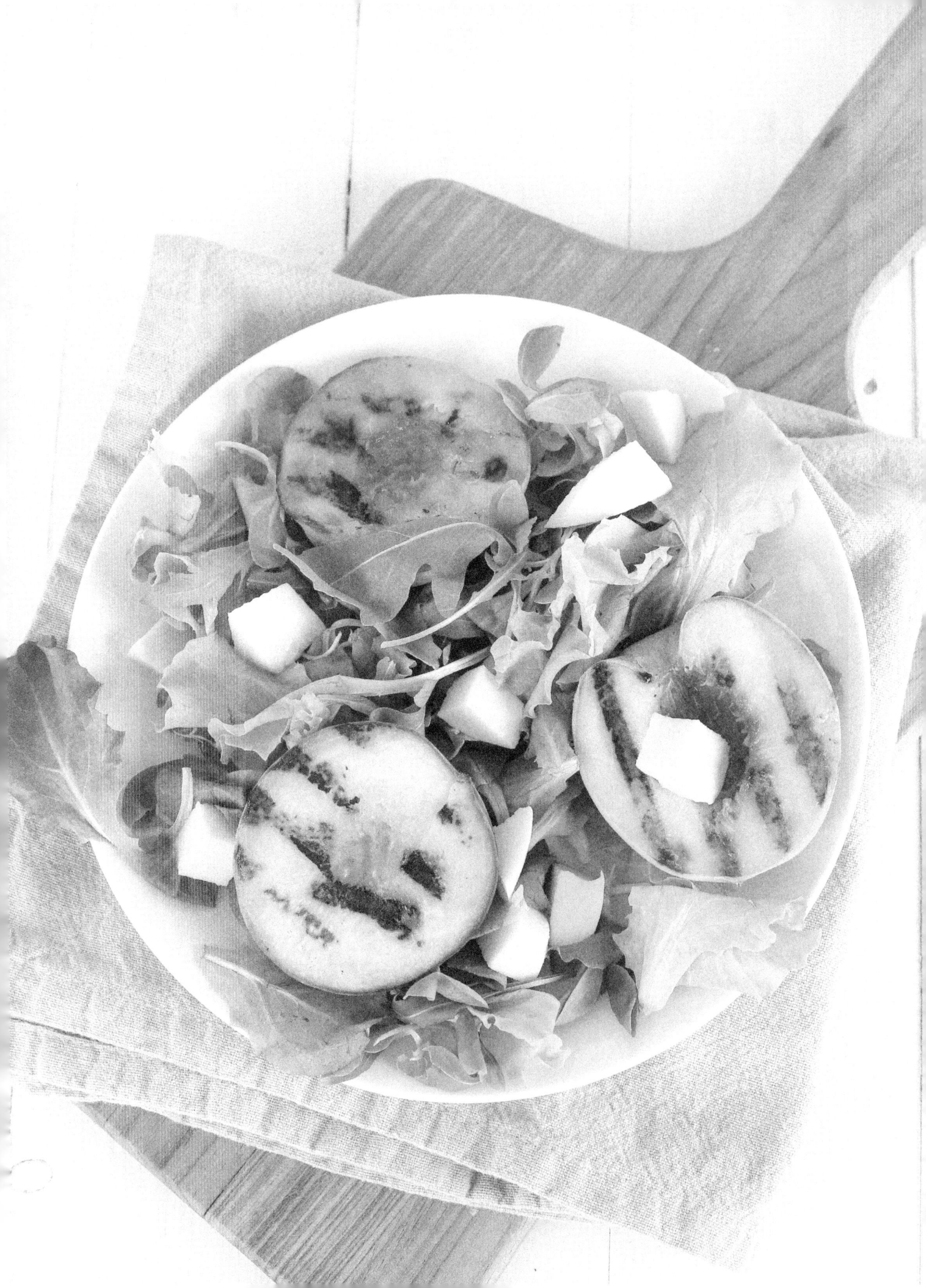

MINT BASIL GRIDDLED PEACH SALAD

SERVINGS - 2

TIME - 15 mins

 NUTRITIONAL VALUE

- Calories-143 kcal
- Carbohydrates-16.7g
- Proteins-1.3g
- Fats-17.8g

 INGREDIENTS

- 1 tbsp lime juice
- 1 tsp lime zest
- 1 tbsp olive oil
- 2 tbsp finely chopped mint
- 2 tbsp finely chopped basil
- 2 quartered peaches
- ¾ cup fine beans
- 1 small red onion
- 1 large lettuce
- 1 avocado

 INSTRUCTIONS

1. Griddle the peach slices on both sides on a pan.
2. Boil up beans on medium flame and set them aside.
3. In a bowl add chopped basil, chopped mint, chopped red onion, sliced lettuce, sliced avocado, olive oil, lemon juice, and lemon zest along with grilled peach slices and serve.

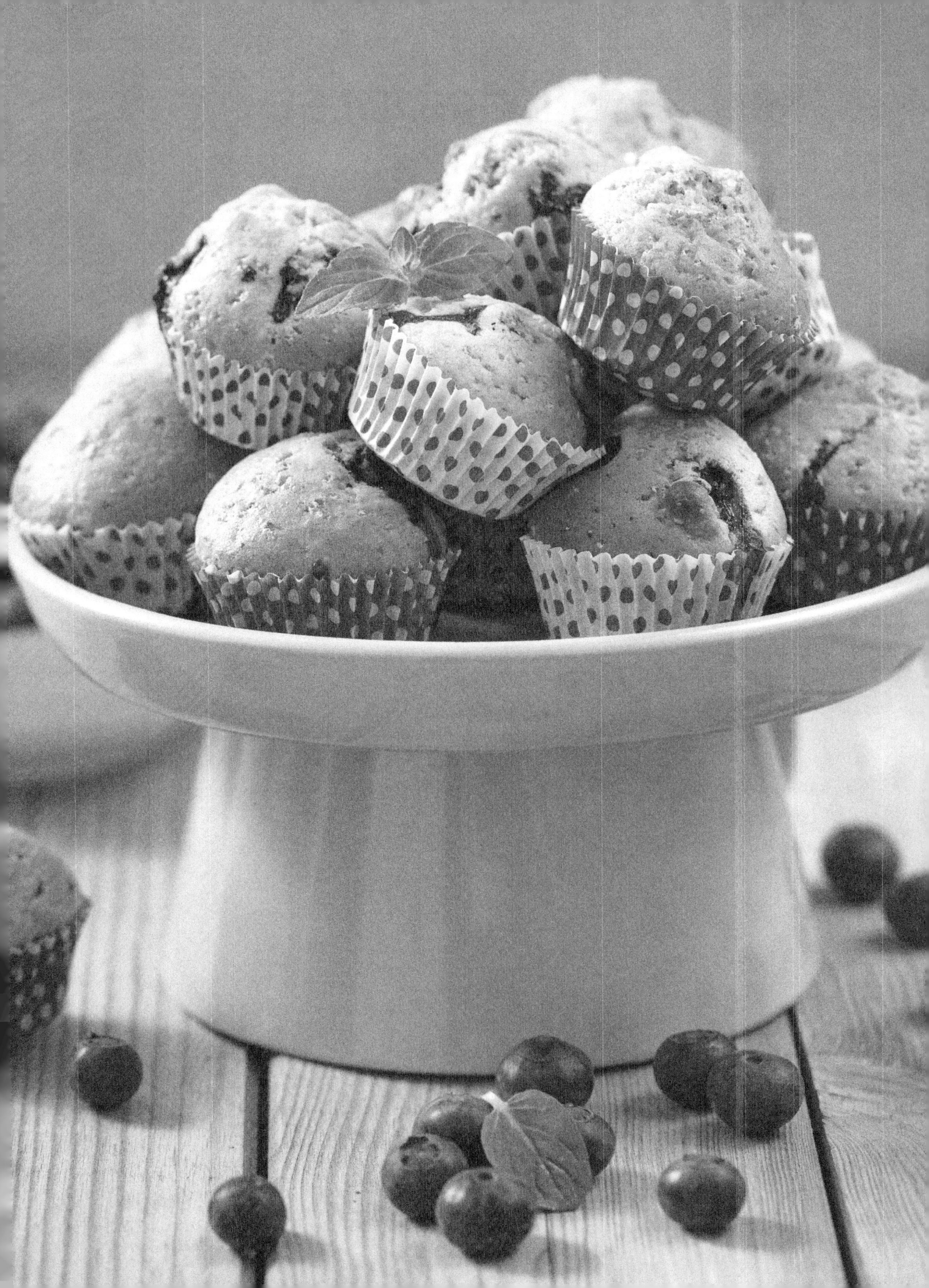

BLUEBERRY MUFFINS

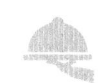

SERVINGS - 12

TIME - 5 mins

 NUTRITIONAL VALUE

- Calories-279 kcal
- Carbohydrates-44.5g
- Proteins-5.4g
- Fats-14.6g

 INGREDIENTS

- 4 cups wheat flour
- 6 tsp baking powder
- 1/3 cup honey
- 1 tsp salt
- 3 tbsp olive cut into slices
- 2 cups blueberries
- 2 eggs
- ½ cup olive oil
- 2 cups non-dairy milk

 INSTRUCTIONS

1. In a bowl add wheat flour along with some salt and baking powder. Set it aside this is your dry mixture.
2. In another bowl whisk eggs together with some honey, milk, and oil.
3. Mix in some blueberries along with some olive slices and combine dry and wet mixtures.
4. Preheat your oven to about 400 degrees Fahrenheit (200 degree Celsius).
5. Grease the muffin tray with some oil and line it with a muffin liner.
6. Add one scoop of mixture in each muffin liner and bake for 18 minutes.

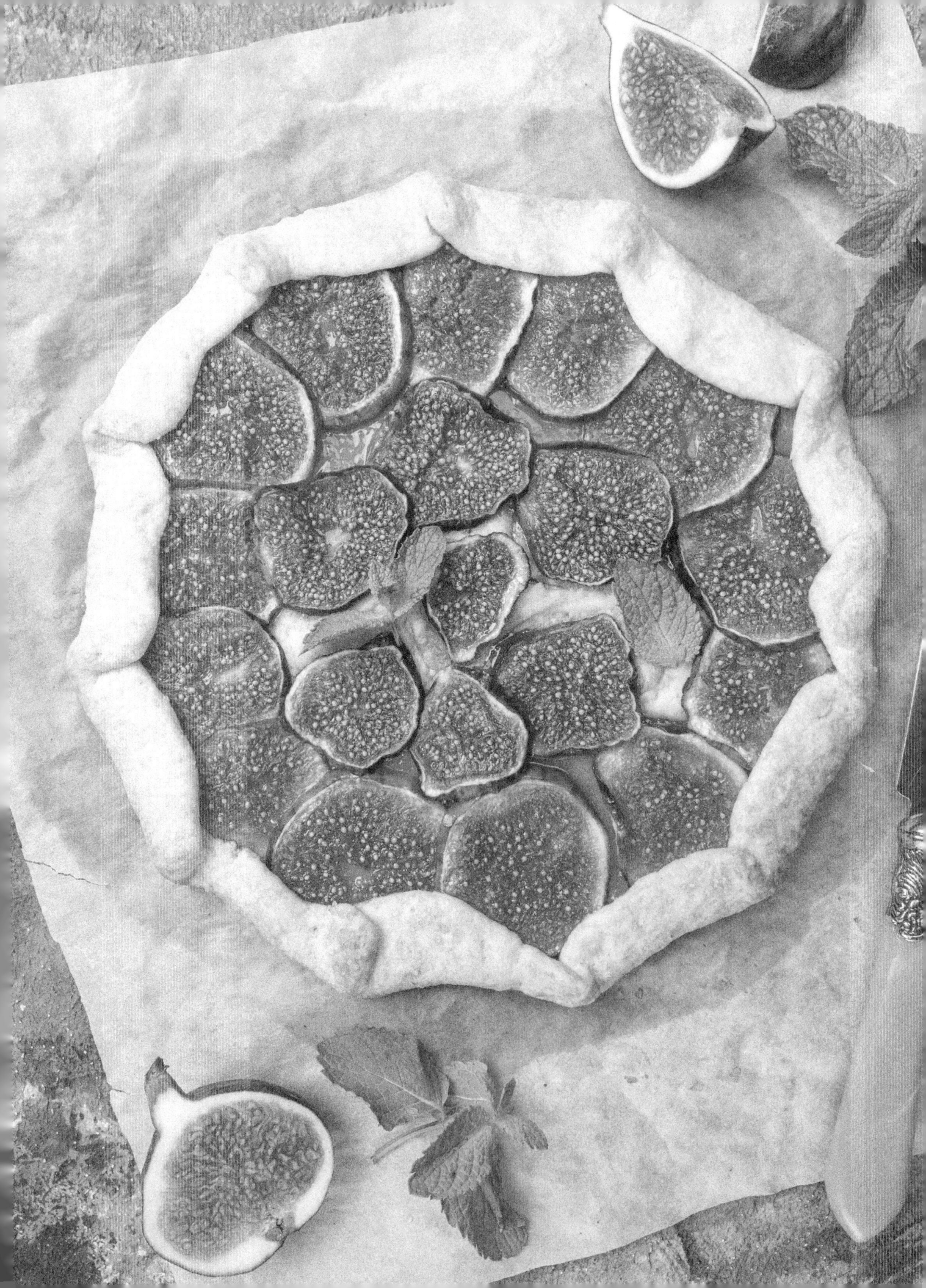

FIG ALMOND OLIVE CAKE

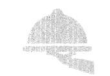

SERVINGS - 5

TIME - 40 mins

NUTRITIONAL VALUE

- Calories-412 kcal
- Carbohydrates-42.4g
- Proteins-6.9g
- Fats-19.6g

INGREDIENTS

- 2 tbsp lemon juice
- 1 tsp lemon zest
- ¼ cup honey
- ¼ cup olive oil
- 2 large eggs
- Salt as per taste
- 1 ½ cup almond flour
- ¾ cup chopped almonds
- 1 ½ tsp baking powder
- 10 fresh sliced figs

INSTRUCTIONS

1. Preheat oven to 350 degrees Fahrenheit (176 degree Celsius). Line up cake mold with parchment paper after greasing it.
2. In a mixing bowl add lemon juice, lemon zest, honey, olive oil, eggs, and salt and mix them well.
3. Fold in some almond flour along with some baking powder and whisk everything well.
4. Drop the batter into the cake mold and drizzle some chopped almonds onto the tray. Bake it for 35 minutes.
5. Cut average slices out of it and enjoy the sweet taste.

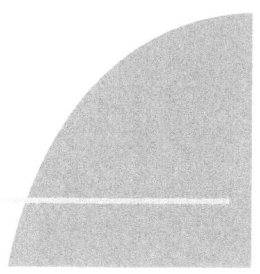

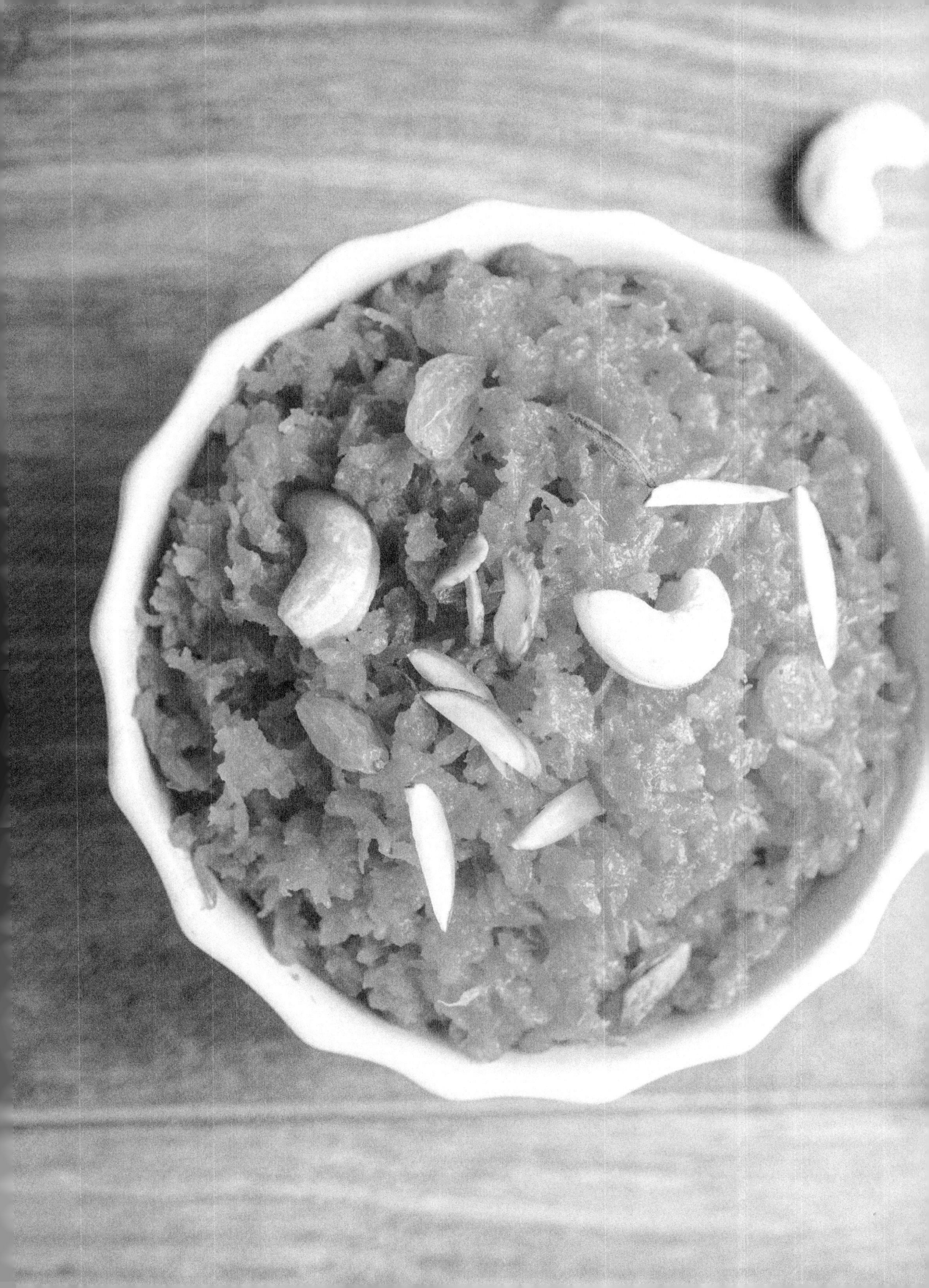

CARROT PUDDING

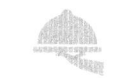

SERVINGS - 2

TIME - 15 mins

 NUTRITIONAL VALUE

- Calories-249 kcal
- Carbohydrates-33.6g
- Proteins-7.4g
- Fats-12.7g

 INGREDIENTS

- 2 cups shredded carrots
- 1 cup non-dairy milk
- 2 tbsp maple syrup
- ¼ cup chopped nuts

 INSTRUCTIONS

1. Take a saucepan and add shredded carrots into it along with some non-dairy milk.
2. Now add maple syrup into it and stir the mixture until carrots are cooked and somehow united with non-dairy milk.
3. Cook it until the mixture gets thickened.
4. At last top up your pudding with some chopped nuts and enjoy when the pudding gets chilled.

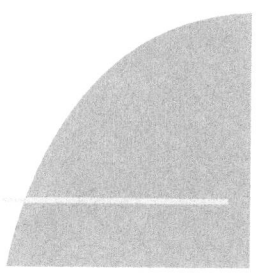

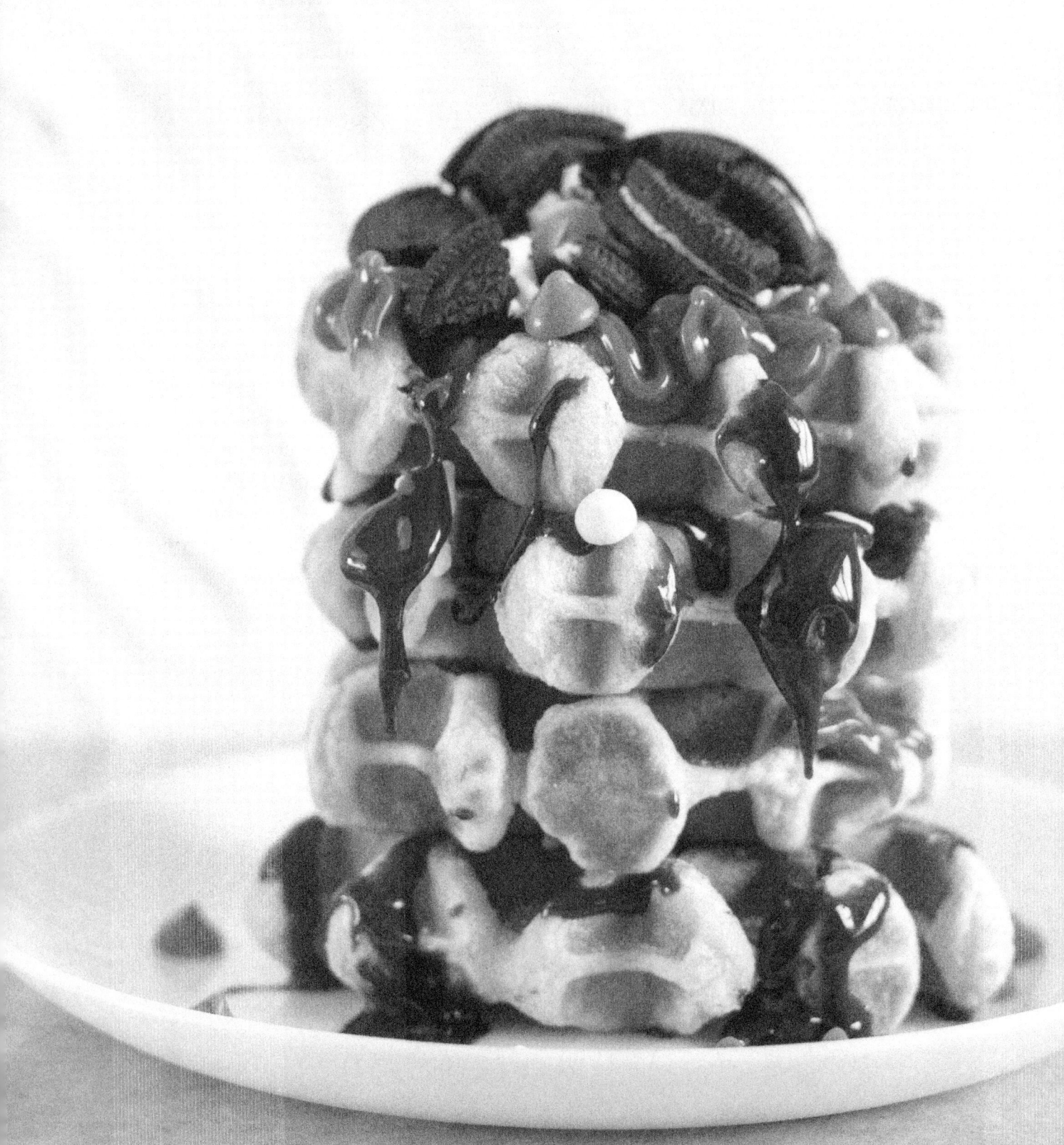

MUSICIANS DESSERT

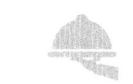
SERVINGS - 2

TIME - 10 mins

NUTRITIONAL VALUE

- Calories-587 kcal
- Carbohydrates-72.5g
- Proteins-13g
- Fats-33.3g

INGREDIENTS

- ¼ cup hazelnuts
- ¼ cup pine nuts
- ¼ cup almonds
- ¼ cup walnuts
- ¼ cup dried apricots
- 1 tbsp raisins
- ½ cup figs
- ½ cup prunes

INSTRUCTIONS

1. Mix all the ingredients in the bowl and enjoy the mixture.

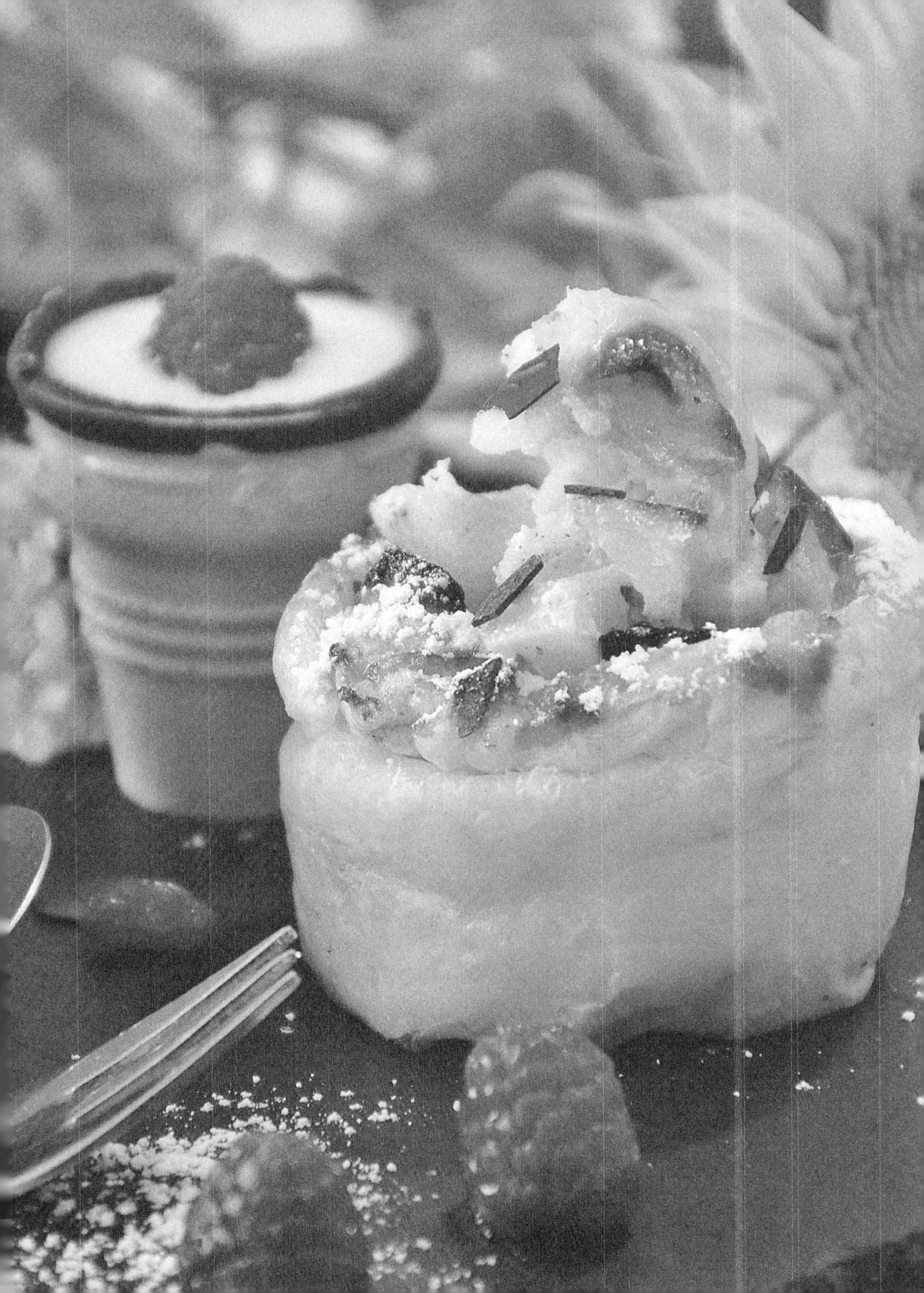

ALMOND DESSERT

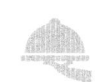

SERVINGS - 4

TIME - 15 mins

 NUTRITIONAL VALUE

- Calories-266 kcal
- Carbohydrates-28.3g
- Proteins-12.2g
- Fats-12.8g

 INGREDIENTS

- 4 eggs
- 2 cups water
- ½ cup brown sugar
- 1 cinnamon stick
- ½ cup ground almonds
- 1 lemon zest
- 2 cups milk

 INSTRUCTIONS

1. Beat egg yolks together with the help of a whisk.
2. Take a saucepan and add water along with some cinnamon sticks, milk, and brown sugar. Bring the mixture to boil and simmer it for 3 minutes to form the golden syrup.
3. Finally, add almonds and lime zest and stir the mixture to form a thick mixture.
4. Cool it and enjoy it once it gets chilled.

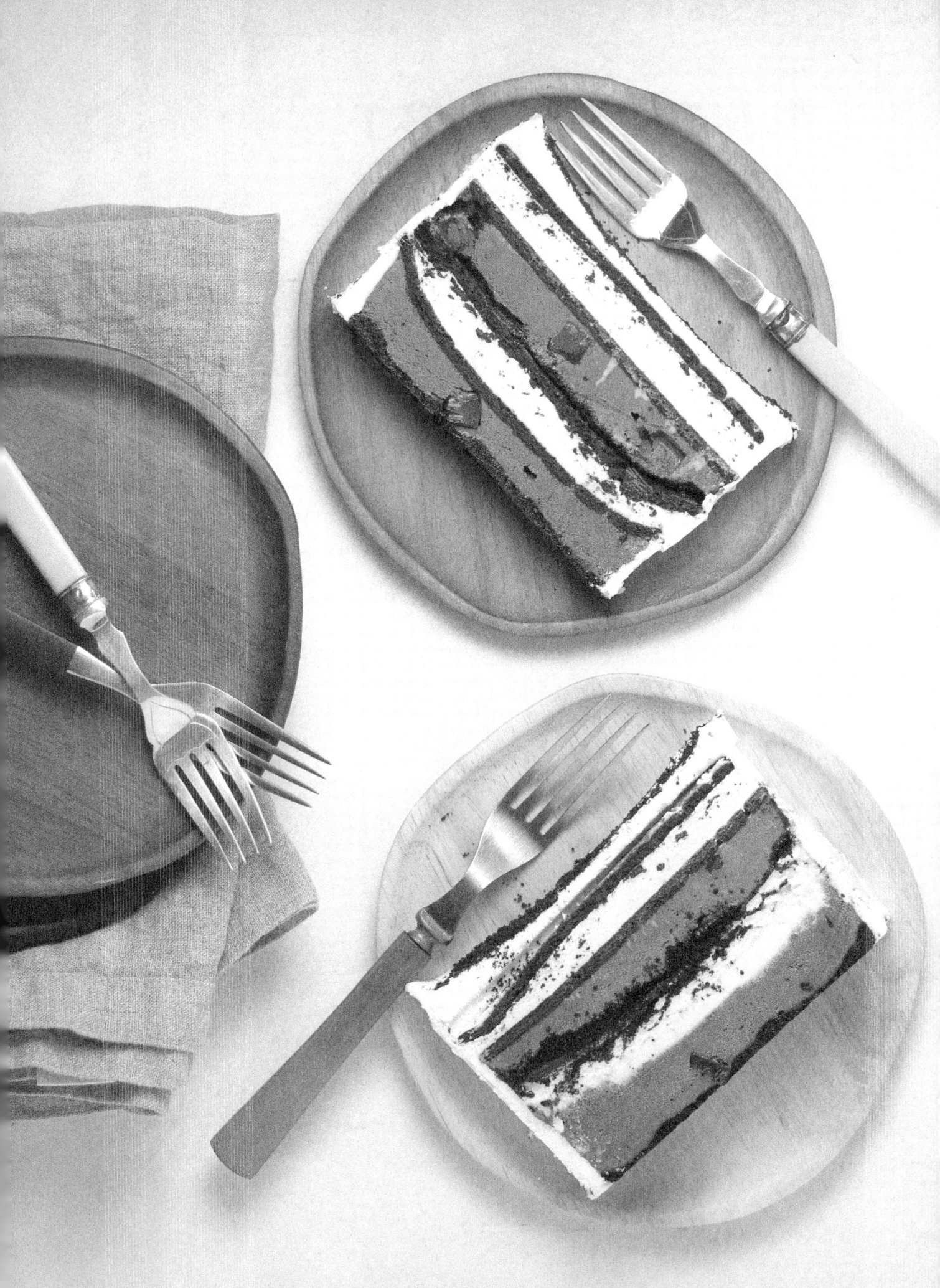

ICE CREAM SANDWICH DESSERT

SERVINGS - 4

TIME - 5 mins

 NUTRITIONAL VALUE

- Calories-309 kcal
- Carbohydrates-57.6g
- Proteins-3.4g
- Fats-7.2g

 INGREDIENTS

- 2 scoops of Raspberry Sorbet
- 4 graham crackers
- 2 tbsp chopped nuts

 INSTRUCTIONS

1. Take two graham crackers and sandwich one scoop of sorbet in between the graham crackers along with some chopped nuts in between.

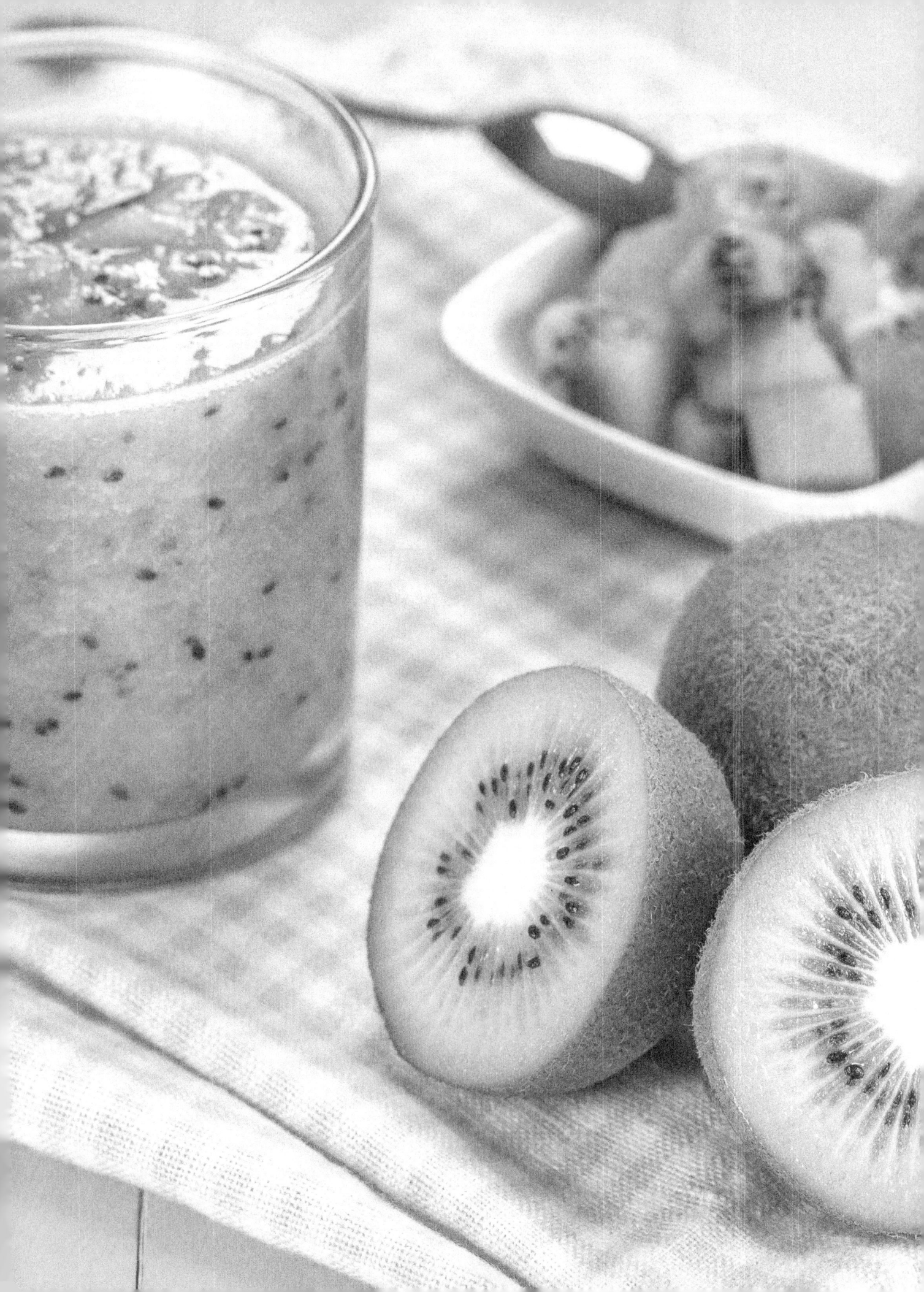

COLD KIWI CREAM DESSERT

SERVINGS - 4

TIME - 10 mins

NUTRITIONAL VALUE

- Calories-212 kcal
- Carbohydrates-39.6g
- Proteins-8.7g
- Fats-2.3g

INGREDIENTS

- 4 kiwi
- 1 cup plain yogurt
- 1 tbsp honey

INSTRUCTIONS

1. In a food processor add yogurt, kiwi, and honey. Blend all the ingredients to form a puree.
2. Place the fruit puree in a container and refrigerate it overnight.
3. Scoop out the dessert and serve with some fresh kiwi slices.

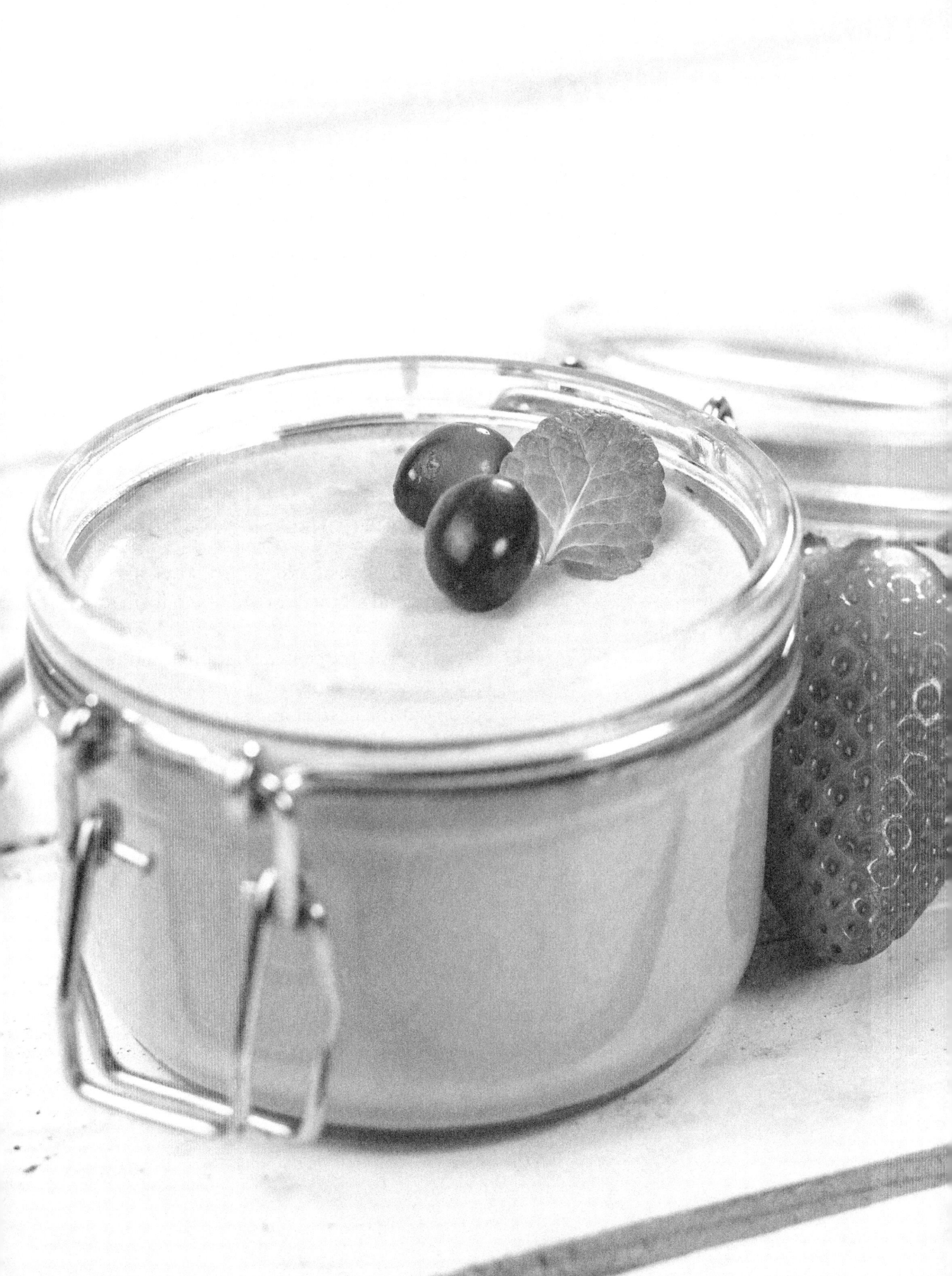

STRAWBERRY MOUSSE

SERVINGS - 4

TIME - 20 mins

 NUTRITIONAL VALUE

- Calories-209 kcal
- Carbohydrates-9.8g
- Proteins-4g
- Fats-19g

 INGREDIENTS

- 1 cup frozen strawberries
- 1 cup vegan cream cheese
- 2 tbsp agar agar
- 1 tbsp cold water
- 2 tbsp erythritol (keto sweetener)

 INSTRUCTIONS

1. First of all puree your frozen strawberries into a mixer or blender.
2. Strain your puree with help of a strainer to get rid of seeds of strawberry and attain a smooth textured puree. Scoop it out in another bowl
3. Next, take vegan cream cheese and put erythritol into it and blend for a smooth texture again
4. Take agar-agar and dissolve it in water and keep it aside.
5. In a vegan cream cheese, bowl add agar-agar mixture and strawberry puree also and give it a nice whisk to homogenize the mixture.
6. Keep it a while so that the mousse might get set.
7. With the help of a piping bag, pipe your strawberry mousse into your serving glass with a garnish of strawberry chunks or slices in-between or on top.

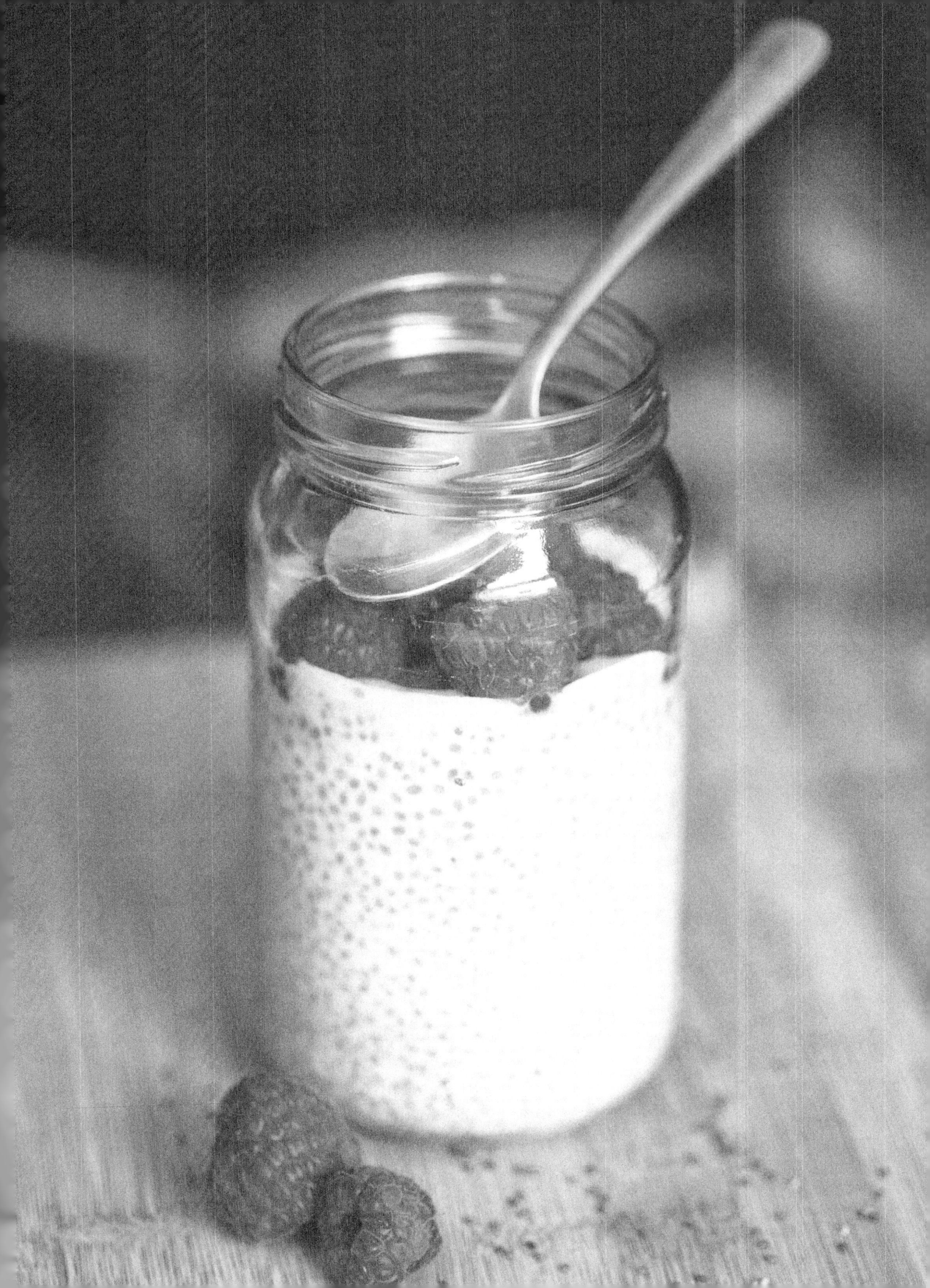

GLUTEN-FREE RASPBERRY ICEBOX PIES IN A JAR

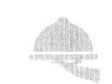

SERVINGS - 3

TIME - 20 mins

 NUTRITIONAL VALUE

- Calories-646 k cal
- Carbohydrates-27.8g
- Proteins-19g
- Fats-53.3g

 INGREDIENTS

- 2 cups raspberries
- ½ cup walnuts
- ¾ cup almond flour
- 2 tbsp brown sugar
- 8-ounce cream cheese
- ½ cup milk

 INSTRUCTIONS

1. Wash raspberries and freeze them until they cool enough
2. In separate baking dishes add walnuts and almond flour and roast them in the oven until aromatic
3. Take a saucepan and add half almond flour and milk in it and cook until the milk gets thickened
4. Take a jar and add roasted walnuts and remaining almond flour at the bottom
5. Scoop out a thick milk saucepan and finally topped with frozen raspberries.

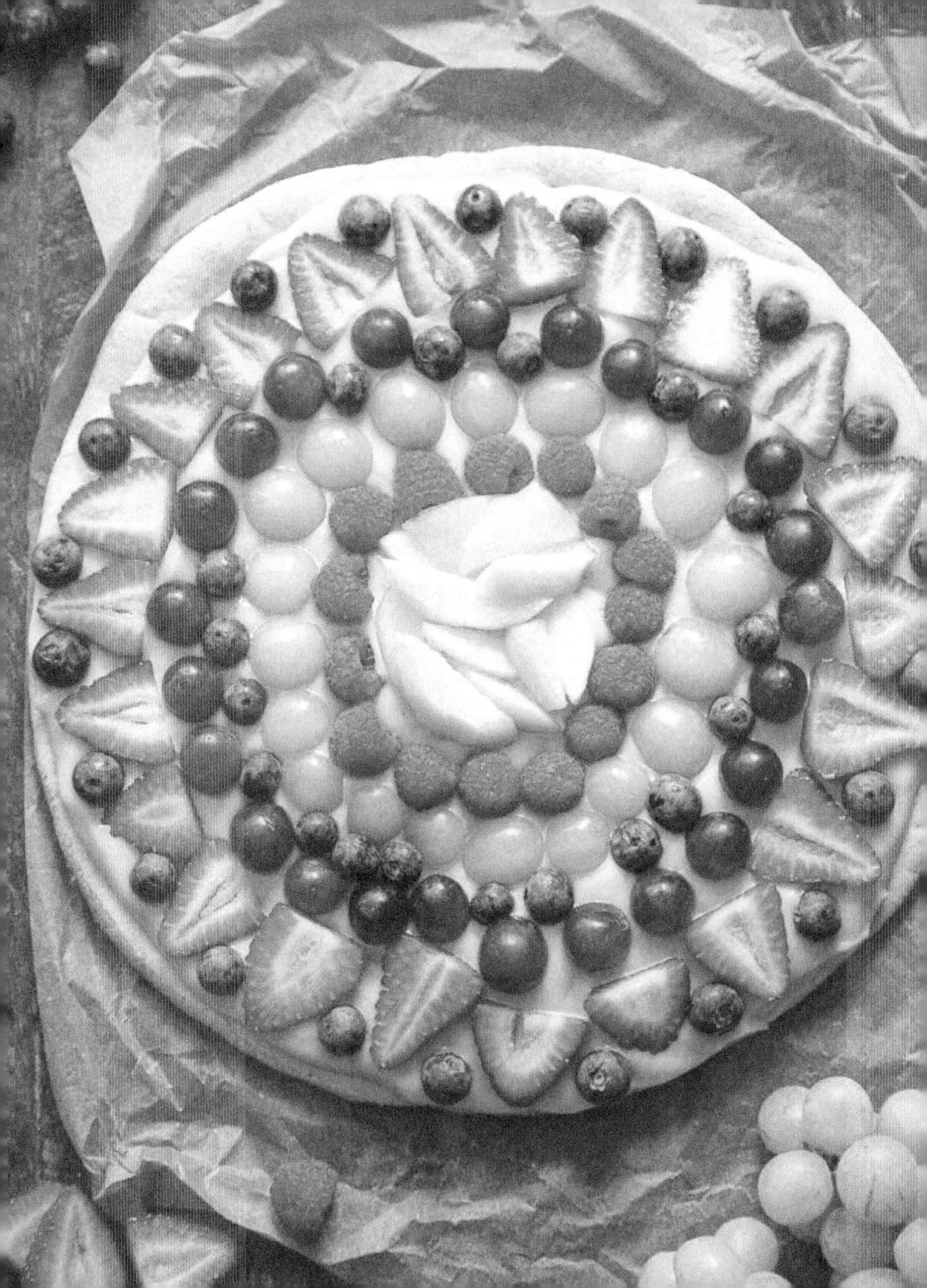

BERRY AND CASHEW CREAM DESSERT PIZZA

SERVINGS - 8

TIME - 30 mins

NUTRITIONAL VALUE

- Calories-339g
- Carbohydrates-27g
- Proteins-6.7g
- Fats-16.5g

INGREDIENTS

Cashew cream:
- 1 cup raw cashews – soaked overnight
- 1 tbsp maple syrup
- 3 tbsp water
- ½ tsp vanilla extract
- 3/4 tsp cinnamon powder
- Pinch of sea salt

Granola Crust
- 1 ½ cup rolled oats
- 1/3 cup shredded coconut
- 1 ½ tsp cinnamon
- ¼ tsp salt
- ½ cup almond butter
- 2 tbsp maple syrup
- 1 tsp coconut oil
- ¾ tsp almond extract
- Fruits
- Blueberry
- Blackberry
- Strawberry
- Raspberry

INSTRUCTIONS

1. For the cashew cream, add all the ingredients including cashews, water, salt, maple syrup, vanilla extract, and cinnamon into a blender and blend until a creamy mixture is formed. If the consistency seems to be thick just add a little bit more water.
2. Preheat oven to to 340 degrees Fahrenheit (172 degree Celsius).
3. In a bowl add rolled oats, shredded coconut, salt, and cinnamon, and mix it well. Your dry mixture is ready.
4. In another bowl, add almond butter, maple syrup, coconut oil, and almond extract. Combine ingredients well. Your wet mixture is ready.
5. Now mix dry mixture into the wet mixture and combine well to form a dough. Now take an 11-inch baking pan and spread the dough onto the greased baking tray. Bake it for 10 to 12 minutes until light golden brown and cool.
6. Spread cashes cream onto the crust and tops it with different varieties of berries.

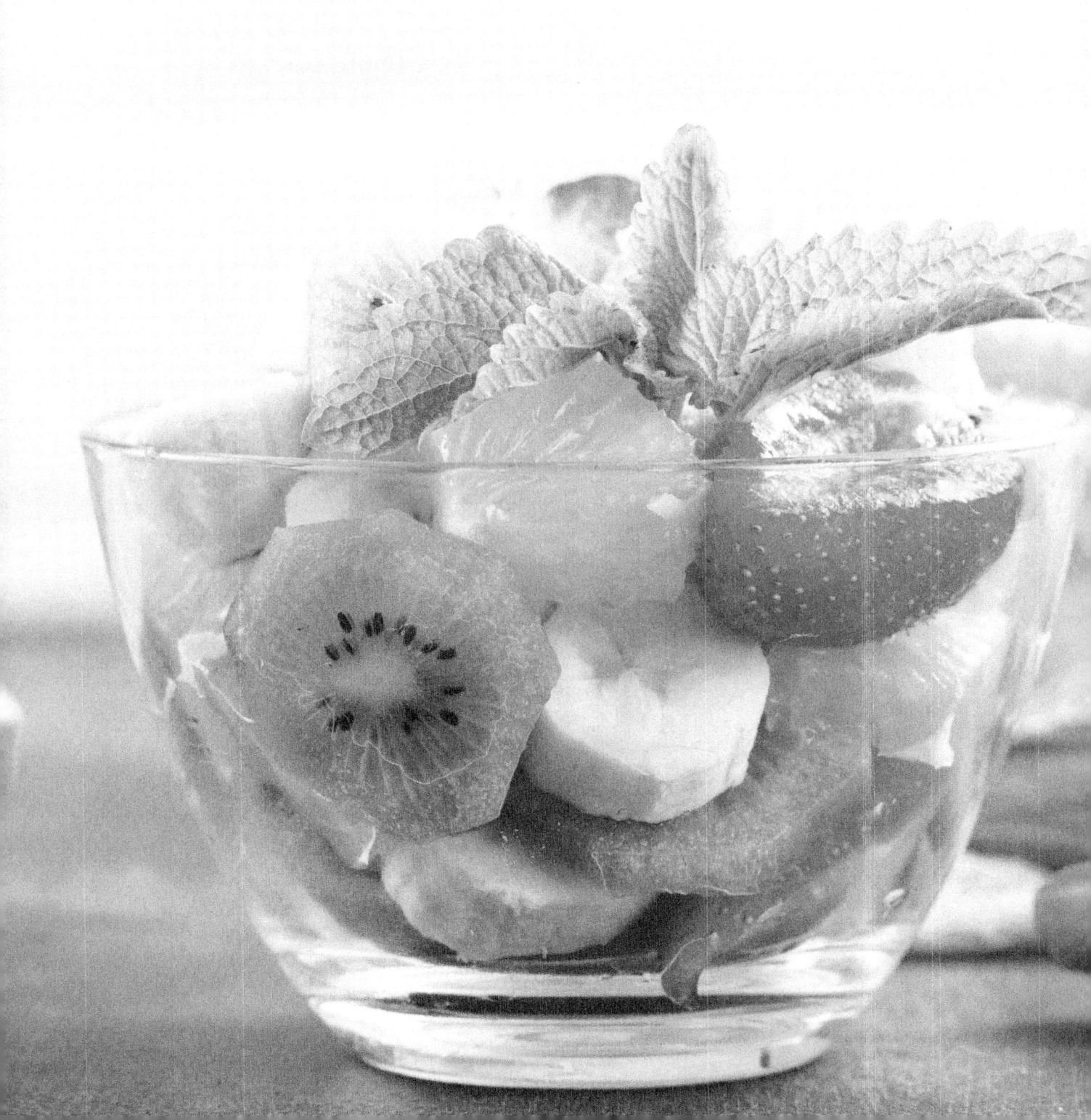

MIMOSA FRUIT SALAD

SERVINGS - 4

TIME - 10 mins

 NUTRITIONAL VALUE

- Calories-157 kcal
- Carbohydrates-37.5g
- Proteins-3.6g
- Fats-4g

 INGREDIENTS

- 1 cup blackberries
- 2 cups kiwi
- 2 cups watermelon
- 1 cup strawberries
- ½ cup orange juice
- Few mint leaves

 INSTRUCTIONS

1. Cut watermelon and kiwi into a large bowl and add strawberries and blackberries in to
2. Take a small bowl and add chopped mint leaves and orange juice for dressing.
3. Drizzle the dressing onto the salad bowl and serve fresh.

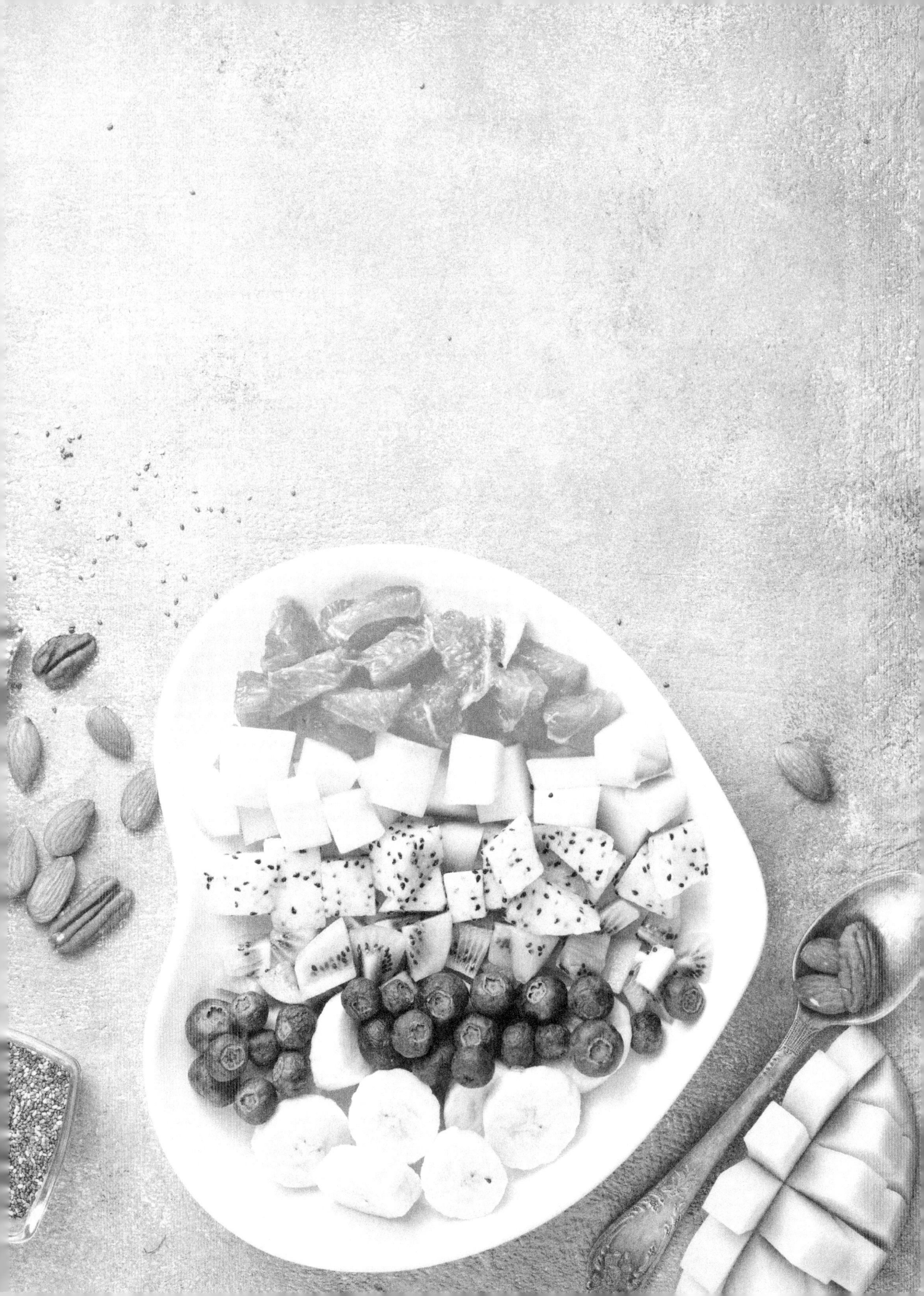

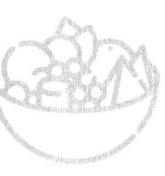

LOW FAT FRUIT SALAD

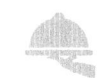

SERVINGS - 4

TIME - 10 mins

 NUTRITIONAL VALUE

- Calories-255 kcal
- Carbohydrates-72g
- Proteins-4g
- Fats-3g

 INGREDIENTS

- 3 sliced bananas
- 4 black grapes
- 2 slices papaya
- 4 strawberries
- 1 diced mango
- 1 diced kiwi
- ½ cup yogurt
- 1 diced apple
- 1 diced pear
- 1 tbsp lemon juice

 INSTRUCTIONS

1. To prepare dressing add bananas, lemon juice, and yogurt into a blender.
2. Add the remaining fruits into a bowl and drizzle some dressing onto the diced fruits.

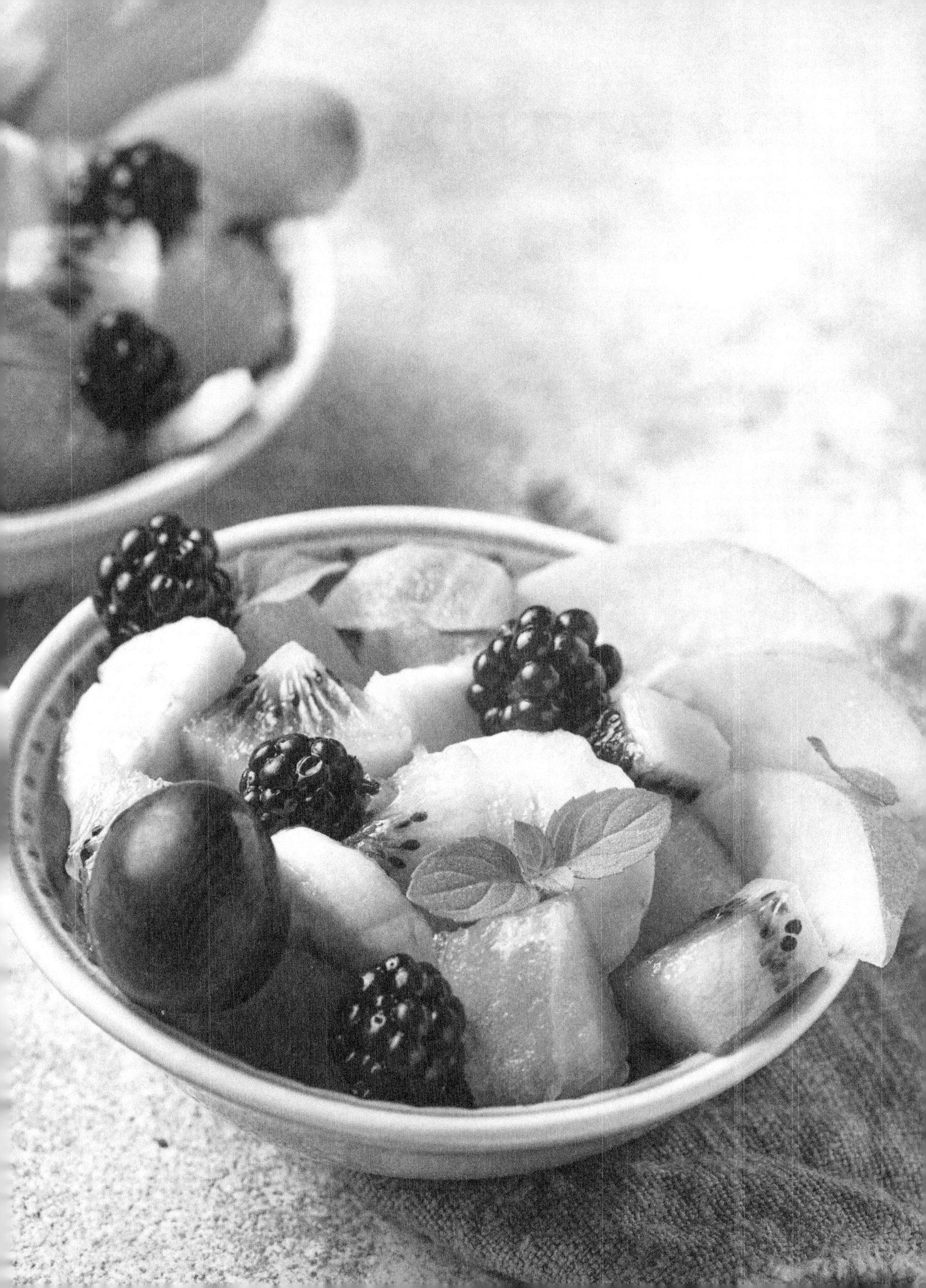

HEALTHY FRUIT SALAD WITH MINT CITRUS DRESSING

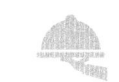

SERVINGS - 4

TIME - 10 mins

NUTRITIONAL VALUE

- Calories-85 kcal
- Carbohydrates-15g
- Proteins-1g
- Fats-0g

INGREDIENTS

- 2 clementine
- ½ cup strawberries
- ¼ cup sliced grapes
- ½ cup diced papaya
- ½ cup diced pineapple
- 1 tbsp lemon juice
- 20 mint leaves

INSTRUCTIONS

1. Mix all the ingredients in a large serving bowl and serve when chilled.

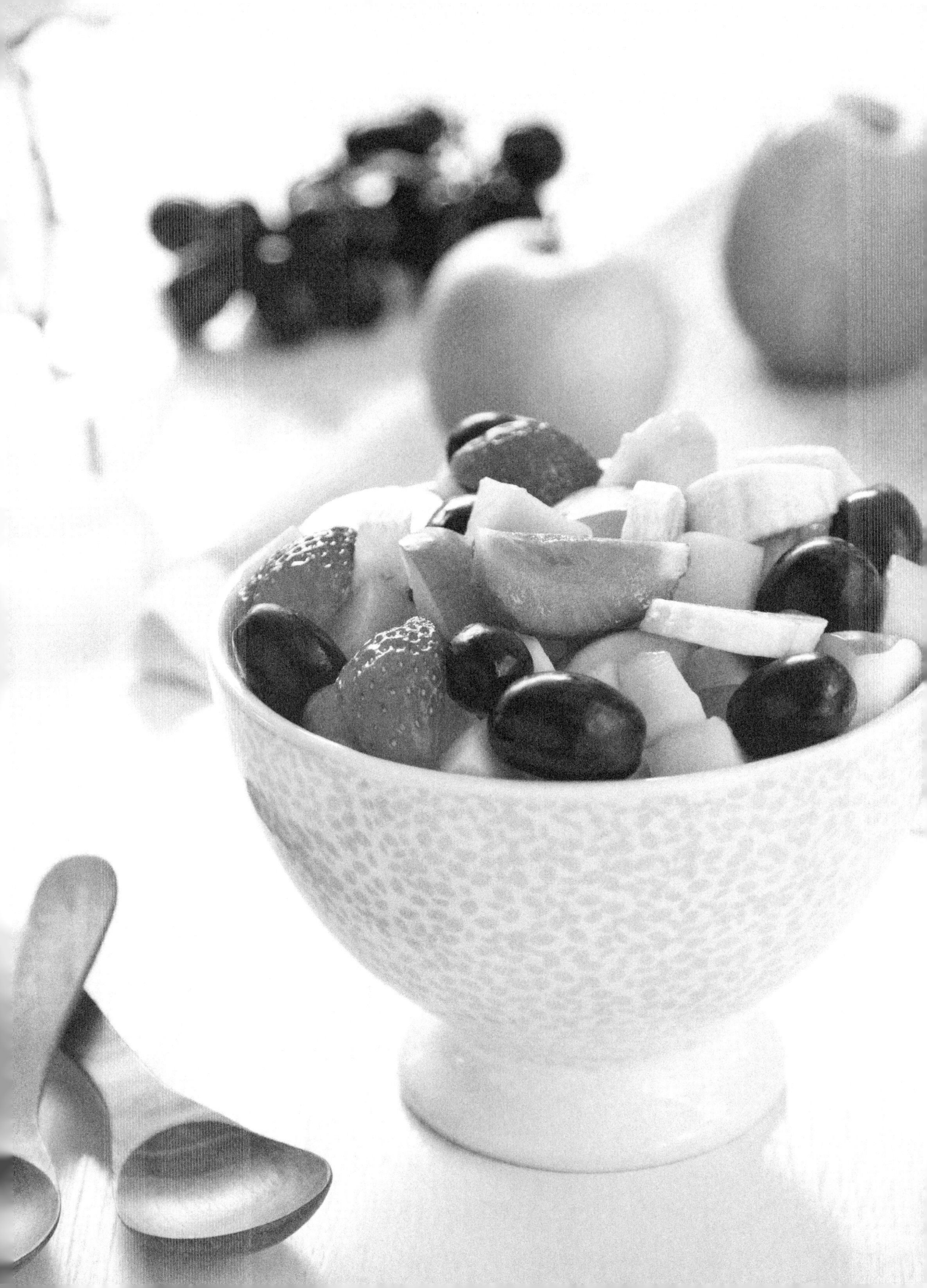

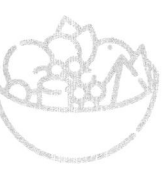

PALEO FRUIT SALAD

SERVINGS - 3

TIME - 15 mins

NUTRITIONAL VALUE

- Calories-246 kcal
- Carbohydrates-62.3g
- Proteins-2.4g
- Fats-0g

INGREDIENTS

- 1 diced apple
- 1 pitted peach
- 1 cup mixed berries
- 2 sliced bananas
- 1 cup grapes
- 1 cup diced pineapple
- 2 tbsp honey
- 1 pinch cinnamon

INSTRUCTIONS

1. Mix everything in a large mixing bowl and serve when chilled.

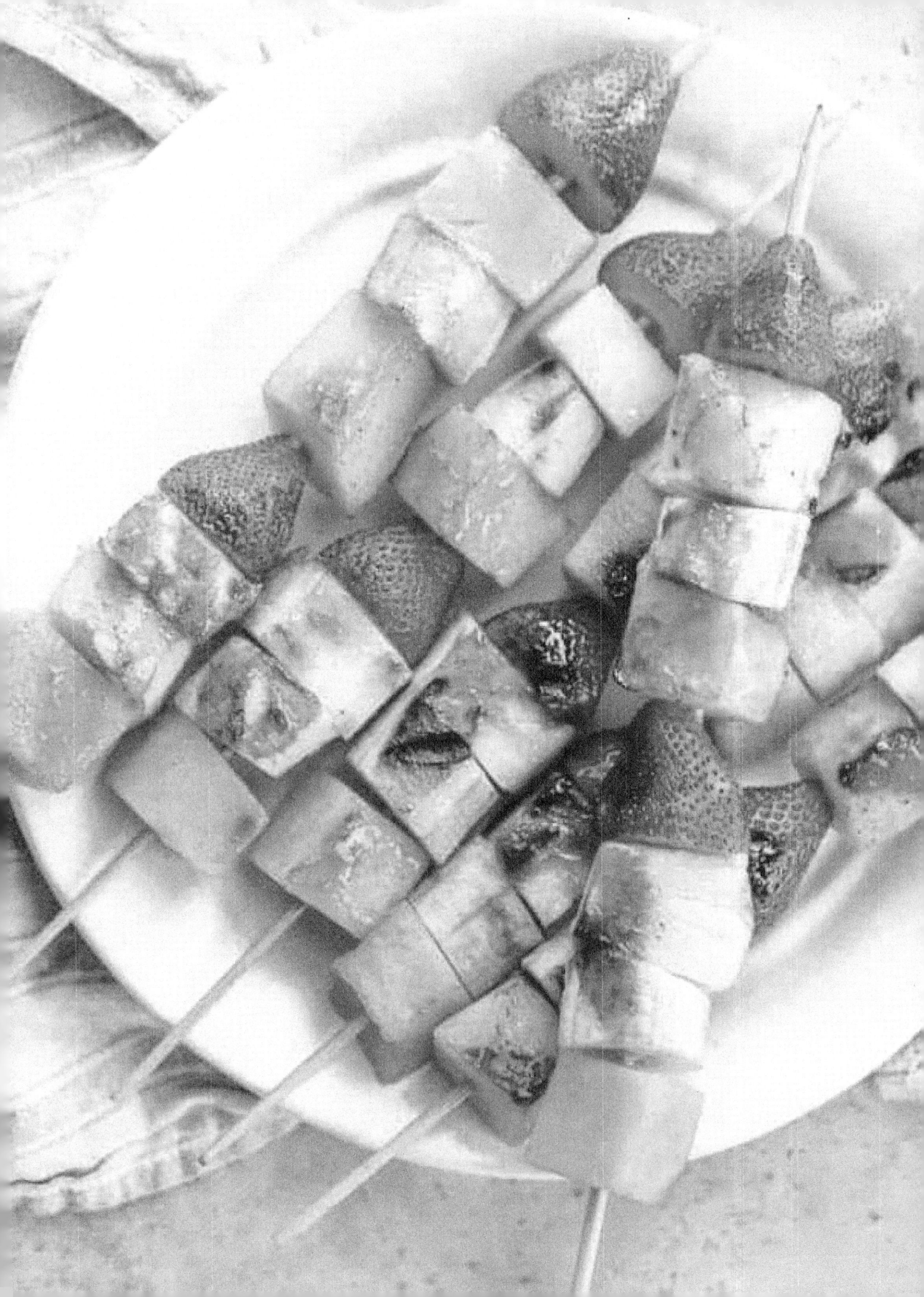

GRILLED FRUIT SALAD WITH COCONUT CREAM

SERVINGS - 4

TIME - 20 mins

 NUTRITIONAL VALUE

- Calories-234 kcal
- Carbohydrates-27g
- Proteins-3g
- Fats-14g

 INGREDIENTS

- 2 tbsp honey
- 1 tbsp lime juice
- 1 cup diced melon
- 1 cup diced mango
- 1 cup strawberries
- 1 tsp coconut oil
- 2 tbsp olive oil
- ½ cup walnuts
- 6 mint leaves
- 6 tbsp coconut cream

 INSTRUCTIONS

1. To prepare coconut dressing, combine coconut cream with honey and lemon juice.
2. Beat the above mixture until cream-like consistency is obtained.
3. Mix all the remaining fruits into the bowl along with some olive oil and coconut dressing.
4. Serve when chilled.

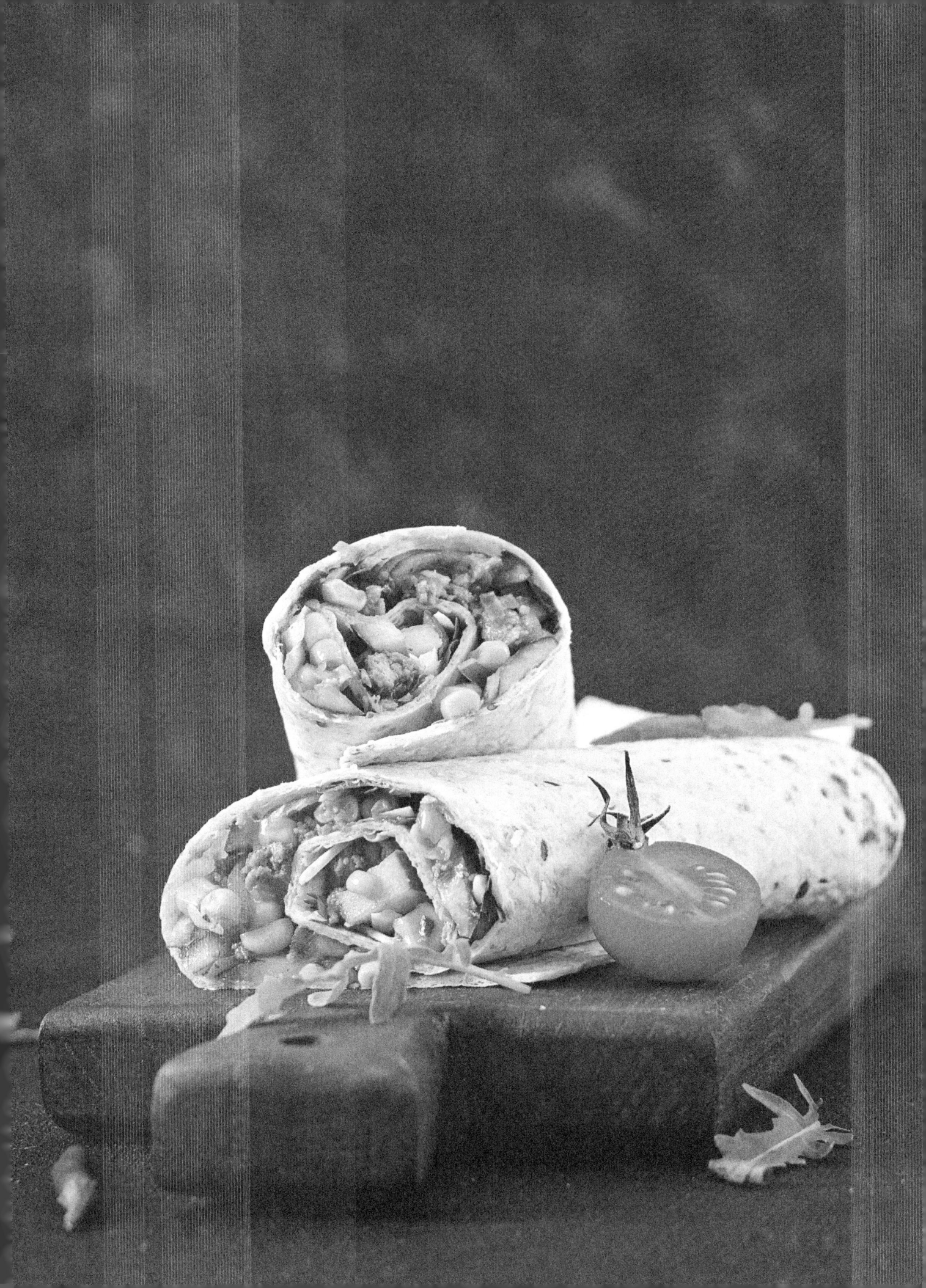

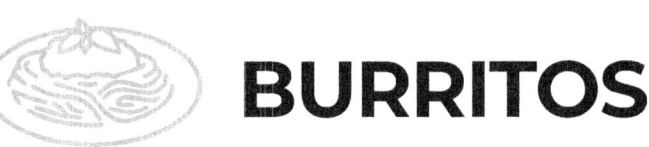# BURRITOS

 SERVINGS - 2

 TIME - 20 mins

 NUTRITIONAL VALUE

- Calories- 614 kcal
- Carbohydrates-6.4g
- Proteins-23.1g
- Fats-52.3g

 INGREDIENTS

- 2 freshly prepared tortillas
- ½ cup tomato salsa
- 3 large eggs
- 1 tbsp almond milk
- Salt as per taste
- Black pepper as per taste
- 1 tbsp olive oil
- 3tbsp sour cream
- ½ cup grated cheese
- ½ sliced avocado

 INSTRUCTIONS

1. Fry tortillas onto a pan. Set it aside.
2. Prepare eggs by adding almond milk to the eggs along with some salt and pepper. Whisk all the ingredients together and cook them into a greased pan.
3. Add cheese onto the tortilla and then add cooked eggs. Also, add some tomato salsa and sour cream, and avocado slices. Roll up tortillas and serve.

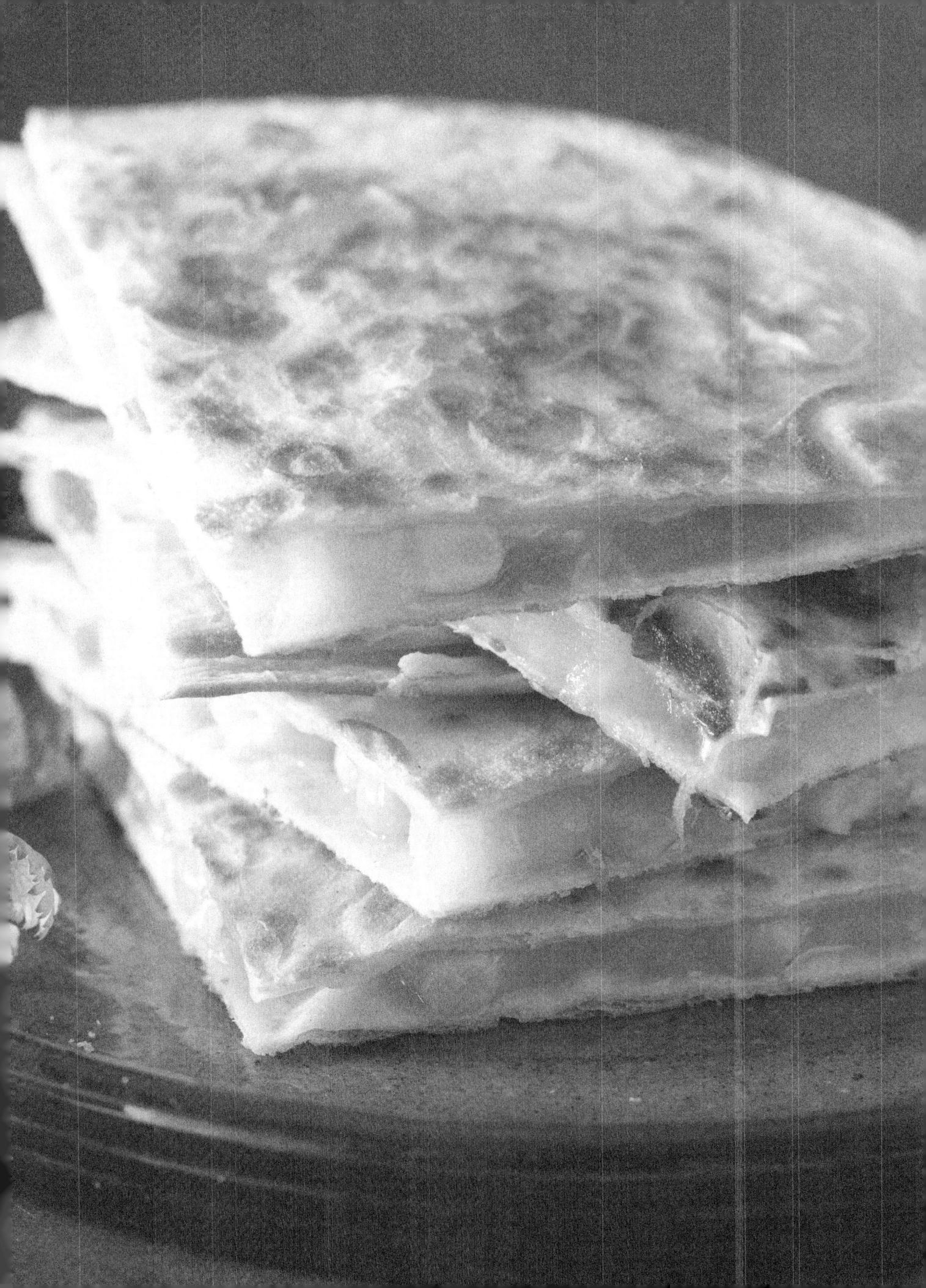

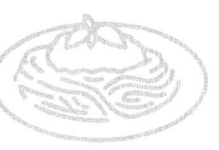

QUESADILLAS

SERVINGS - 2

TIME - 20 mins

 NUTRITIONAL VALUE

- Calories-258 kcal
- Carbohydrates-48.2g
- Proteins-8.3g
- Fats-3g

 INGREDIENTS

- 1 cup wheat flour
- Water as per requirement
- 2 tbsp shredded cheese
- 2 tbsp mix veggie salsa

 INSTRUCTIONS

1. In a mixing bowl add wheat flour and water together. Knead the dough and make small balls out of the dough.
2. Roll out the dough into a tortilla and heat it on a griddle on both sides.
3. Take a tortilla and drizzle some cheese along with some salsa onto it.
4. Wrap the tortilla and enjoy.

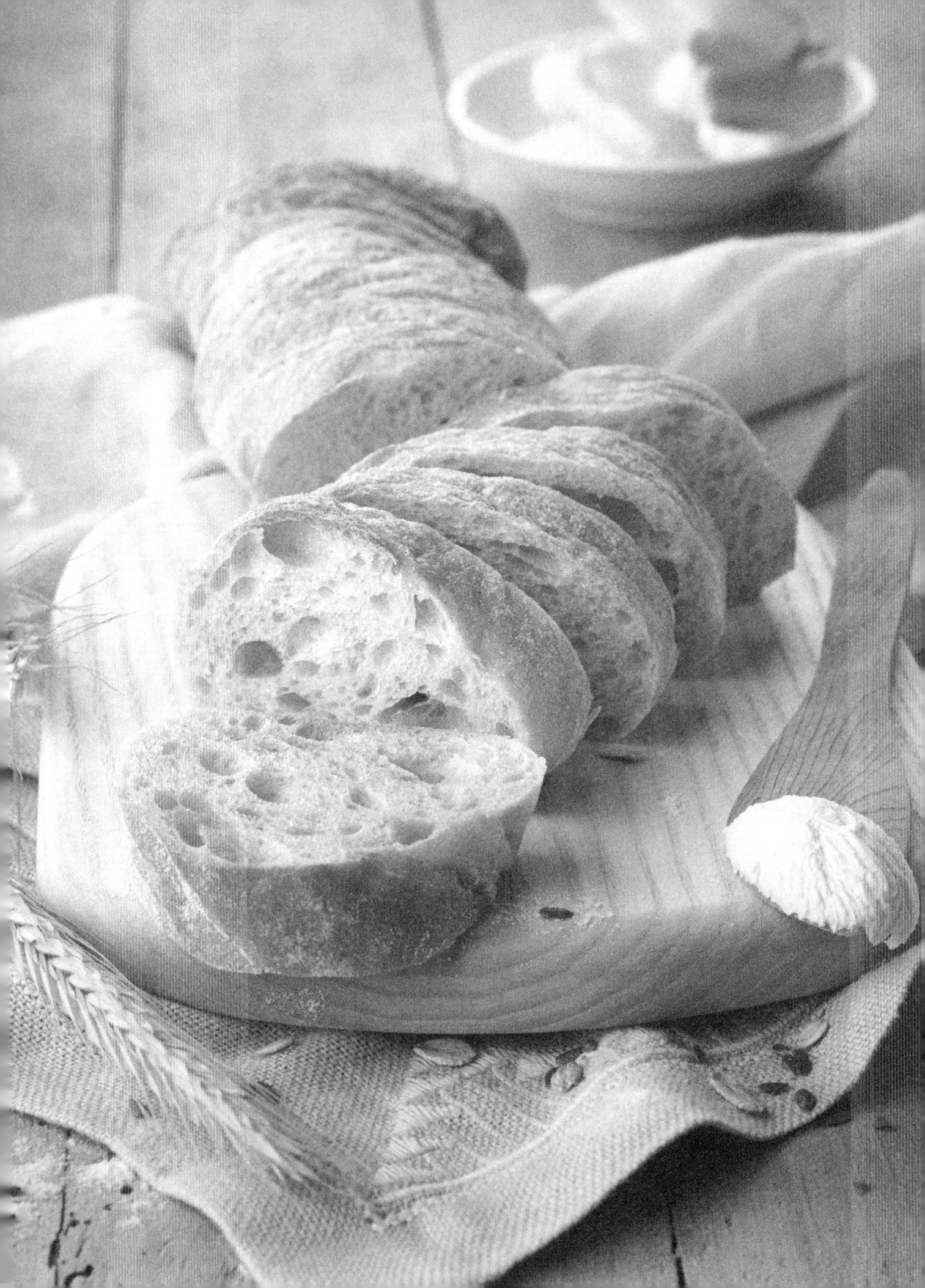

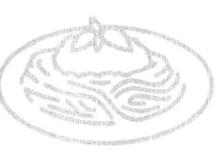

LIGHT BREAD

SERVINGS - 6

TIME - 20 mins

 NUTRITIONAL VALUE

- Calories-165 kcal
- Carbohydrates-2g
- Proteins-6g
- Fats-12g

 INGREDIENTS

- 1/3 cup ground psyllium husk powder
- 1 ¼ cup almond flour
- 2 tsp baking powder
- 1 tsp salt
- 1 cup water
- 2 tsp apple cider vinegar
- 3 egg whites
- 2 tbsp sesame seeds

 INSTRUCTIONS

1. In a large mixing bowl add all the dry ingredients including psyllium husk powder, almond flour, baking powder, salt, and a few sesame seeds.
2. Add egg whites and vinegar to the above mixture and whisk the ingredients together.
3. Then add a bit of boiling water and mix to form a dough.
4. Knead the dough with your hands and by applying the olive oil to your palms make 6 small balls out of the dough.
5. Preheat your oven at 375 degrees Fahrenheit (200 degree Celsius) and place balls on the baking sheet.
6. Bake the bread pieces for 40 minutes and serve with a favorable filling or topping.

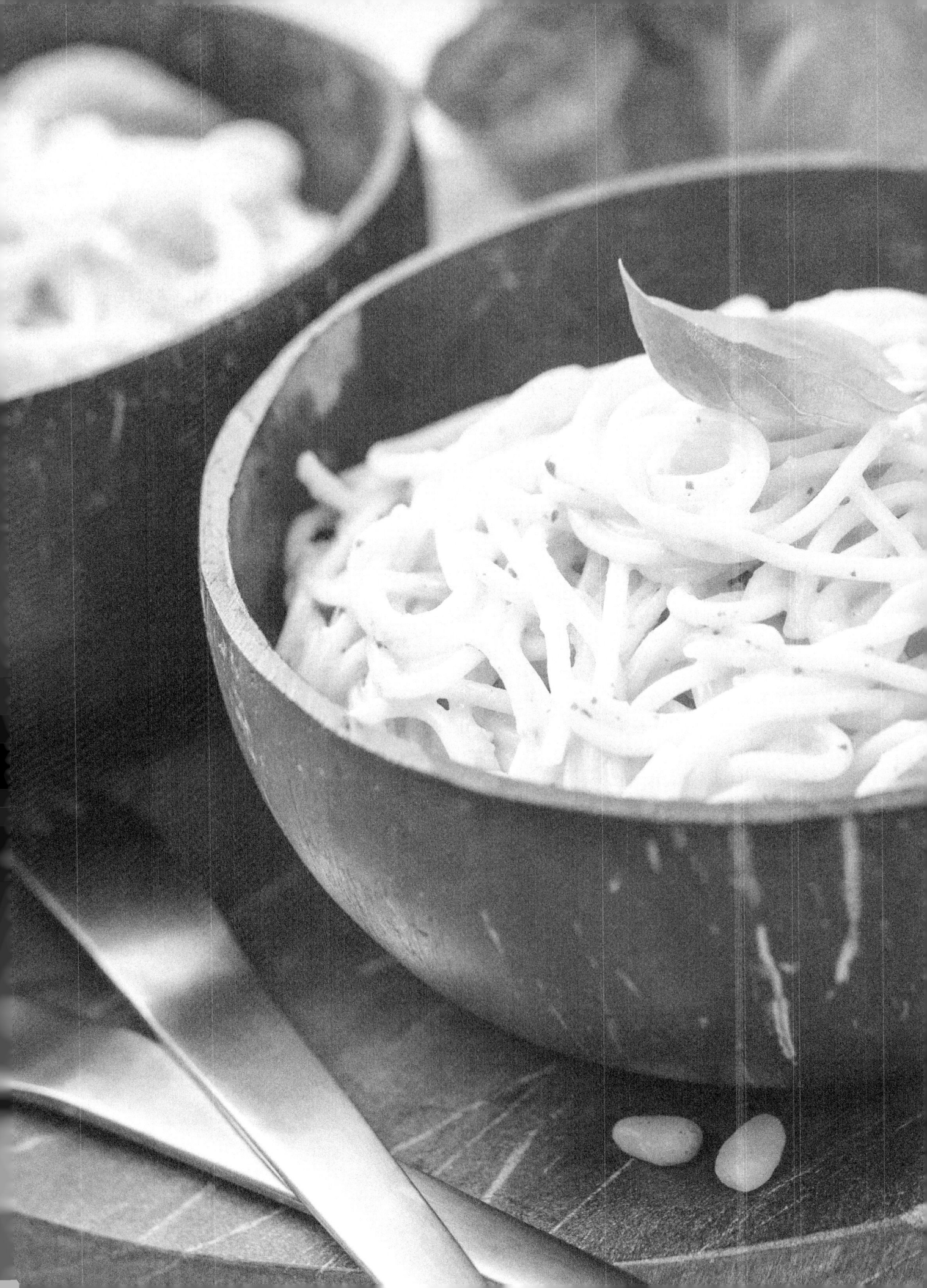

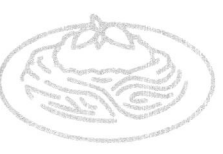

DIET PASTA

SERVINGS - 4

TIME - 20 mins

NUTRITIONAL VALUE

- Calories-240 kcal
- Carbohydrates-34g
- Proteins-3g
- Fats-9g

INGREDIENTS

- 2 cups brown pasta
- 1 cup mixed vegetables
- ½ cup tomato puree
- 1 chopped onion
- 1 tsp black pepper
- 1 tbsp chopped green chilies
- 1 tsp salt
- 1 tsp cumin seeds
- 1 tsp fresh coriander

INSTRUCTIONS

1. Boil pasta and drain it.
2. Take a cooking pan and add oil to it. Sauté some onions into it and add cumin seeds.
3. Add mixed vegetables and stir fry them for few minutes.
4. Also, add tomato puree along with remaining spices.
5. Garnish with chopped chilies and coriander leaves.

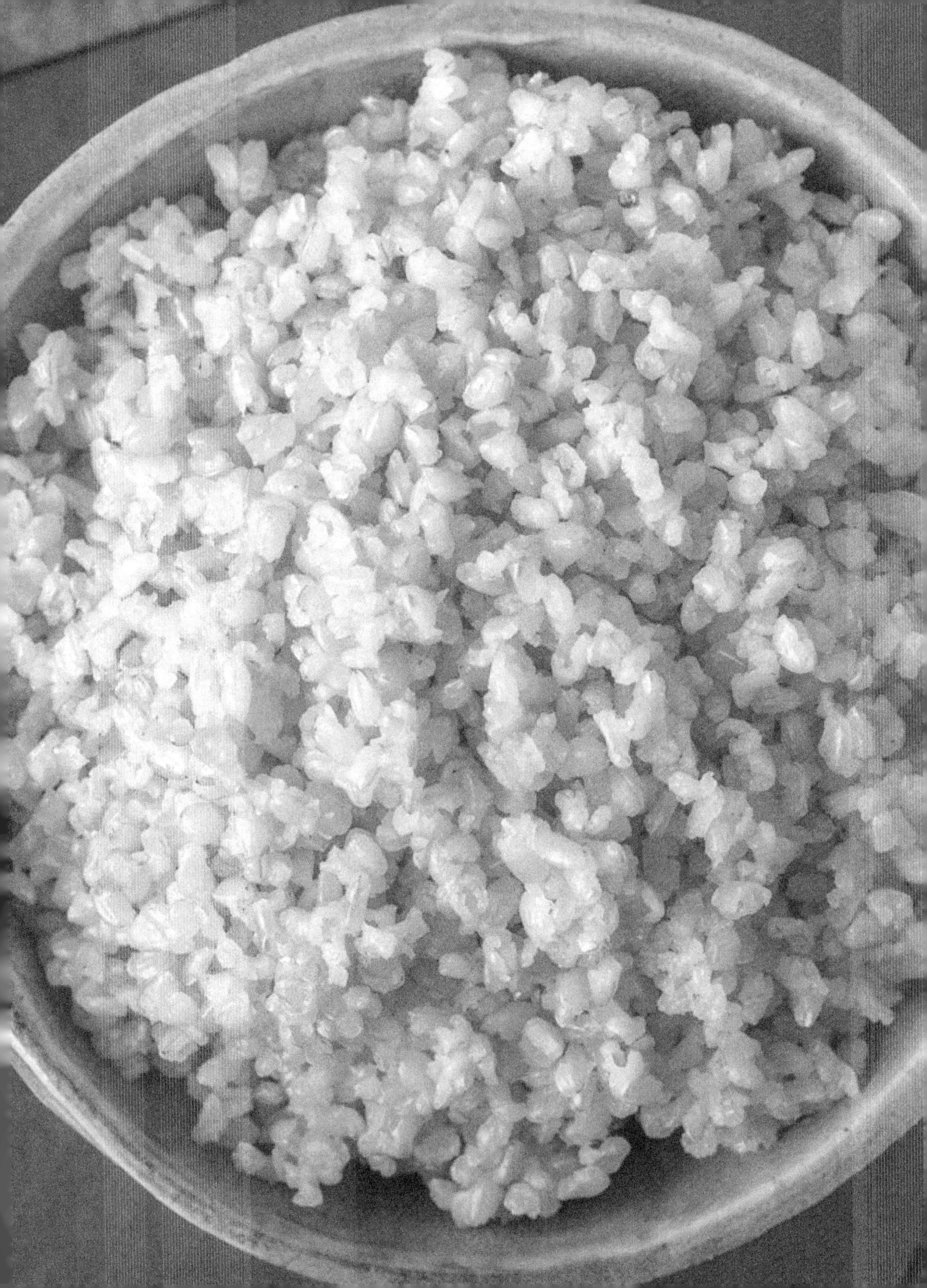

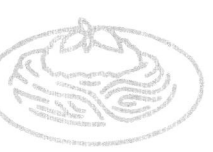

EASY BROWN RICE

SERVINGS - 2

TIME - 20 mins

NUTRITIONAL VALUE

- Calories- 113kcal
- Carbohydrates-24g
- Proteins-2.3g
- Fats-1g

INGREDIENTS

- 2 ½ cup broth
- 1 cup brown rice
- 1 tsp salt

INSTRUCTIONS

1. Boil broth in a pot and add salt to it.
2. Once the broth is boiled add soaked brown rice into it.
3. Wait for 20 minutes on medium flame and serve.

Dear Reader,

I hope you did enjoy the book and are now closer to your goals. I genuinely hope you are and this book helps you.

Would you be open to leaving a review on Amazon? It's cool if you'd prefer not to, but leaving a review will help me understand what my readers like and what they do not like. I assure you that I read all of the reviews and consider them when writing the next book. Just put down a few words about your thoughts. I will very much appreciate it.

I wish you all the best

Danielle De Mayo

Printed in Great Britain
by Amazon